MW01236130

Arthritis: 277 Things Everyone Should Know

A Guidebook For The More Than 40 Million Americans Who Suffer From
Arthritis But Are Committed To Maintaining Their Independence

Wendy Reed Bruce

First Edition

Live Oak Publications Inc., Metairie, Louisiana

Arthritis: 277 Things Everyone Should Know

A Guidebook For The More Than 40 Million Americans Who Suffer From Arthritis But Are Committed to Maintaining Their Independence

By Wendy Reed Bruce

Published by: Live Oak Publications, Inc.
2901 Ridgelake Drive Suite 107
Metairie, LA   70002
U. S. A.

Copyright © 1998
First Printing 1998

Author: Wendy Reed Bruce
Editor: Peggy Furr
Cover Design: Robert Howard

ISBN   1-891985-00-0

Books are available in quantity for promotional or premium use. Write to Judith Zabalaoui, Live Oak Publications, 2901 Ridgelake Drive Suite 107, Metairie, LA 70002, for information on discounts and terms, or call toll-free 1-888-504-5950.

Table of Contents

> *When in doubt, follow the directions.*

Table of Contents

Keep following the directions.

Preface

I want to congratulate you on "showing up." By opening this book, you have shown that you are not only interested in arthritis, you are willing to do something about it. You are taking an active role—you are becoming a partner in your health. This attitude alone can make a tremendous difference in dealing with the disease. And that is, after all, the goal of this book—to better equip arthritis sufferers to deal with their chronic condition.

Good Luck!

—Wendy Reed Bruce

> "Showing up is 80 percent of life."
>
> —Woody Allen

T o those who know the disease peripherally,

Those who work with it professionally,

But especially, those who live with it personally.

Acknowledgments

Thanks go to—

My support system—Scott, Brittany, Brianne, and Reed; Gramba and Grandaddy for "Reed-sitting" during this project; Shelia Goodwin, my informative physical therapist and cousin; and the Birmingham Chapter of the Arthritis Foundation.

Where to Go for Help:

The Arthritis Foundation is unparalleled in its assistance to arthritis sufferers. Call (800) 283-7800 for your local chapter and area services.

Medical:

Definitions

Statistics

Symptoms

Drug Therapy

Surgery

Arthritis is not one disease. It's actually the term used to refer to over 120 different diseases associated with the joints. Literally translated, arthritis means joint inflammation—"arthro" is the Greek word for joint and "itis" means inflammation. It should be noted, however, that inflammation is not always present. A truer definition might be "problems usually associated with the joint(s) but which can also affect the muscles and connective tissues of the body, including the skin and the organs."

———

Breaking down words will help you understand medical terminology. Sometimes medical terms seem foreign and frightening simply because they're long. Breaking them down can reveal they are not as complicated as you thought. For example, polyarticular simply means many joints—poly (many) and art (joint). Likewise, monoarticular means one joint—mono (one) and art (joint).

———

Currently, it is estimated that 40 million Americans have arthritis. By the year 2020, that number may increase to almost 60 million. As the baby boomers age, arthritis will affect more people than even cancer, heart disease, or other major health problems.

Medical

Arthritic conditions cause more disability and financial loss than any other chronic illness. Approximately three million people are limited in their everyday activities, such as dressing, bathing, and walking. Approximately 45 million days are lost from work, 156 million days are spent in bed, and 427 million days of restricting activity can be attributed to its effects. Its cost in the U.S. in 1992, including indirect costs, such as lost wages and medical care, is estimated at an incredible $65 billion.

Despite the fact that one in three families and one in seven people are affected, the annual federal investment in research amounts to less than $3 per person, compared with an average of $150,000 per person in cost and care over their lifetime.

Don't despair!!! The outlook is not bleak!!! Major advances in research and treatment are still being made. Some forms of arthritis can be cured, such as septic arthritis, or controlled almost 100 percent, such as gout.

> *Approximately three million people are limited in their everyday activities.*

Arthritis fatigue is real !!!

Inflammation

You would be hard pressed to discuss arthritis without using the word inflammation. You might be harder pressed to define exactly what inflammation is, though. Let me try to explain without speaking "medicalese." Inflammation is the body's protective response to an injury or infection. The classic signs—heat, redness, swelling, and pain—are produced as a result of biochemicals secreted by your body's infection-fighting immune cells as they attempt to destroy germs and remove damaged tissue. Usually once the battle is won, the inflammation subsides. This is not the case with rheumatoid arthritis.

———

Arthritis fatigue is real! Don't let anyone make you think you're just lazy or unmotivated. Fatigue is very likely your body's reaction to substances released into your bloodstream by activated immune cells. Fatigue can be used as a barometer to monitor your current condition when you know your normal fatigue threshold. When you begin to feel fatigued earlier in the day than normal, your condition may be worsening.

Osteoarthritis (OA)

OA is one of the oldest and most common diseases of man. It affects almost 16 million people, most over the age of 45. Once commonly thought of as a "wear- and-tear" disorder, doctors now believe it doesn't have a single cause. It is probably a result of a combination of genetics and joint mechanics, such as misalignment. The likelihood of developing it does increase with age, however. Just ask anyone over 75; chances are they have it.

———

OA is labeled degenerative because cartilage breaks down or degenerates. Cartilage is the slippery smooth, rubbery material that covers the end of each bone. (Think gristle.) Its surface enables the joints to glide smoothly. The breakdown occurs in several phases. First, the smooth cartilage surface loses its elasticity, softens, and becomes frayed. This pitting weakens the cartilage and makes it more vulnerable to injury and damage.

Osteoarthritis was detected in "Ice Man," the name given to a 5,000 year-old mummified body found in the Alps.

> *Osteoarthritis and rheumatoid arthritis can occur at the same time.*

As a result, over time, large sections may be worn away, allowing the bones to rub against one another—OUCH! The joints may then lose their shape and the bones may thicken at the end and form bony growths. Fluid-filled cysts may also form and bits of cartilage or bone may float in the joint space—DOUBLE OUCH! Unfortunately, the cartilage doesn't grow back once it is worn away.

———

OA can affect any joint (It only affects joints, unlike rheumatoid arthritis.), but it most commonly occurs in the hips, knees, and spine. The finger joints, the joint at the base of the thumb, and the joint at the base of the big toe are also frequently affected. Waists, shoulders, ankles, and jaws are rarely affected.

Medical

Common Causes of Osteoarthritis

Heredity

- People may have a defect in the gene responsible for producing collagen, a major component of cartilage.

- People may be born with joint alignment defects, such as bowed legs.

- People may be born with laxity (double jointedness) which also increases their chances

Obesity

- People who are overweight increase the stress their joints must bear.

- People with OA weigh an average 15 pounds above their recommended weight.

Injury

- People who experience a joint injury have a greater chance of developing OA in that joint.

- People who repeatedly use the same joint(s) increase their risk of injury for that joint.

People with OA weigh an average 15 pounds above their recommended weight.

> *Stress is related but does not cause arthritis. Some believe testing for stress-related hormones can predict the course of RA, but it's iffy.*

Rheumatoid Arthritis (RA)

Approximately 6.5 million Americans are afflicted by this mysterious form of arthritis. It is characterized by joint and/or organ inflammation. With joint involvement, a symmetrical pattern is usually observed. That is, if the ring-finger knuckle is swollen on the right hand, the same joint will also be swollen on the left hand. Such inflammation is the result of the immune system—the body's defense against bacteria, viruses, and other foreign cells—going haywire. The immune system mistakenly attacks its body's own tissues and organs. Such a catastrophe in the armed forces is called "friendly fire."

———

Why RA strikes people is unknown; that it can strike anyone is fact. Neither men, women, nor children are spared. It does, however, seem to prefer women three to one over men, and it is more likely to begin during the young to middle adult years.

RA Inflammation

The inflammation of RA can last for extended periods and can cause serious, irreversible damage as a result. This fact necessitates early diagnosis and treatment.

In RA, a defect in the body's immune system causes it to turn renegade and attack its own tissue. White blood cells—the foot soldiers—move from the bloodstream into the joint tissues, resulting in excess fluid. This causes more inflammation, more damage, and a painful cycle begins. Over a period of time, this cycle damages the cartilage and may actually eat away part of the bone. Muscle aches, fatigue, muscle stiffness (especially in the morning), and low-grade fever often accompany the inflammation.

In RA, a defect in the body's immune system causes it to turn renegade and attack its own tissue.

> *RA is a synovial arthritis as is most juvenile arthritis.*

Categories of Arthritis

We've discussed the two types of arthritis that are the most common: rheumatoid arthritis and osteoarthritis. Let's take a quick look at a few of the other 125 forms of this disease.

It is helpful to know that there are eight different categories of arthritis:

➤ The first is known as *synovitis.* This word means that the synovial membrane which creates the joint's lubricating fluid is inflamed. RA is a synovial arthritis as is most juvenile arthritis.

➤ *Enthesopathy* is an inflammation where the ligaments and tendons attach to the bones.

➤ *Microcrystalline arthritis* is a category of arthritis where tiny crystals form in the joint space itself, creating swelling and pain.

- ➢ *Joint infections* are the fourth category. Bacteria or other germs get in the joint fluid and create an arthritic inflammation.

- ➢ The fifth category is *cartilage degeneration.* This is the category of osteoarthritis (OA).

- ➢ *Muscle inflammation* is the sixth category of arthritis. This is an unusual form.

- ➢ *Local conditions* usually result from local problems like irritation or injury, but not from disease. Technically, this may not be arthritis, but if not properly treated, can lead to it.

- ➢ *General conditions* involve aching and stiffness throughout the body.

General conditions involve aching and stiffness throughout the body.

> *Lupus is considered an autoimmune disease where the body's own antibodies attack it as if they were attacking a virus.*

Other Kinds of Arthritis

Within the synovial category, we find *Lupus (Systemic Lupus Erythematosus, SLE)*. Lupus is considered an autoimmune disease where the body's own antibodies attack it as if they were attacking a virus. Only about half the people who have lupus have arthritis. It is not usually as severe as RA although the joints affected are commonly the same ones that are involved in RA. Symptoms are pain and tender joints. The prognosis is ordinarily good for this type of arthritis.

———

Ankylosing spondilitis (AS) is an arthritis that is categorized as enthesopathy. Most of the sufferers seem to be men, with onset typically between ages 15 and 40. The most noticeable aspect of AS is a "poker spine" where the back becomes very stiff and unable to bend because the bones fuse together. AS is a genetic disease and tends to occur in families. It is especially prevalent among North American Indians and is very rare among blacks. It is most frequently a mild condition and not usually a serious problem. Motion exercise is used to delay or prevent fusion.

The most common form of microcrystalline arthritis is *gout*. Gout is a very painful arthritic condition where uric acid crystallizes in the joint space causing a throbbing illness. Increased uric acid in the blood leads to the formation of gout crystals. There is now very satisfactory drug treatment for patients with gout and no significant problem with health should result from it. Because gout is affected by body weight, diet, and alcohol, it can be managed even without drug therapy.

———

A much more serious form of arthritis under the category of infection is the possibility of a *staphylococcus* or *staph* infection of the joint space. A single "hot joint" is an emergency and needs immediate attention. If not properly and quickly treated, it can lead to complete destruction of the joint and, at worst, death. This form of arthritis can be cured by antibiotics, but immediate treatment is essential to prevent joint destruction. Other joint infections can be caused by *gonococcus,* the bacteria that causes gonorrhea, or by the *tuberculosis* bacterium.

> *Gout is a very painful arthritic condition where uric acid crystallizes in the joint space, causing a throbbing illness.*

> **Bursitis will usually heal within a week to ten days.**

*P*olmyalgia rheumatica (PMR) is categorized under muscle inflammation. PMR has been recently recognized as a major form of rheumatism. It causes muscle pain and consequent restriction of movement, usually in the neck and shoulder regions, as well as the hip area. The average age of onset is about 70. It can come on suddenly or gradually. Morning stiffness may accompany it. Sufferers may be tired, have a low fever, and lose weight. The most serious possible effect is loss of vision in one or both eyes. However, when treated with a corticosteroid like Prednisone, most people respond marvelously within a day or two.

———

*C*arpal tunnel syndrome, *frozen shoulder*, and *tennis elbow* are some of the arthritic conditions categorized as local. *Bursitis* is another. Bursitis is an inflammation of the *bursa* which is a small sac of tissue containing a lubricating fluid that eases the movement of muscle across muscle or muscle across bone. Inflammation of this sac results in localized pain. It can be the result of injury, repeated pressure on the area, or overuse. Bursitis will usually heal within a week to ten days. Rest, warmth, a sling, gentle range-of-motion exercises, time, and avoidance of the injury-causing activity are the best antidotes. See your doctor if the discomfort persists.

Medical

General conditions of aching and tenderness all over are included as arthritic-type conditions because the symptoms are so bothersome for sufferers, especially when long-term. *Fibromyalgia, psychogenic rheumatism,* and *depression and arthritis* fall into this category. Fibromyalgia is the most common of these syndromes, affecting as many as five million people in the United States. Its symptoms include aching in many parts of the body, abnormal sleep pattern with morning stiffness and fatigue, and specific points of tenderness on the body. Fibromyalgia does not result in deformity, but it can be very distressful and disabling for the sufferer. Treatments include exercise and, sometimes, drugs.

Some forms of arthritis can involve unpredictable fatigue that can affect a person's quality of life.

> *Arthritis was the dominant cause of activity restraint among American women from 1989 through 1991.*

Women and Arthritis

Arthritis is the most commonly experienced chronic disease among older women. It was the dominant cause of activity restraint among American women from 1989 through 1991.

———

The risk of having arthritis increases with age and weight. For women age 65 and older, the rate of arthritis was 55.8 percent, 33.5 percent for women ages 45 through 64, and 8.6 percent for women ages 15 through 44.

———

Arthritis was more prevalent in women with annual incomes under $10,000.

———

The incidence of arthritis among women is expected to increase to 35.9 million by 2020.

Primary care physicians can direct and coordinate arthritis treatment. If therapy from any other specialist is required, the primary care physician will make a referral.

Rheumatologists specialize in treating rheumatic diseases. They generally treat the more complicated forms of arthritis. Most patients with mild to moderate cases don't require a rheumatologist.

Physical therapists use non-drug methods to relieve pain and inflammation based on patients' individual needs. These include muscle strengthening, range-of-motion and endurance exercises, water therapy, and relaxation techniques.

Occupational therapists help patients go about everyday living—dressing, working, cooking, etc.—by teaching new ways of performing these activities.

Registered nurses are a link between doctor and patient. They can be helpful in answering day-to-day questions.

More Specialists

in Arthritis Care

Social workers aid with the social, emotional, and financial concerns associated with arthritis. They can help determine what benefits a patient is eligible for, assist in getting job counseling, and provide guidance to appropriate programs.

Mental health counselors help patients cope with the emotional problems and stressful conditions that may result.

Physiatrists are medical doctors who specialize in the physical rehabilitation of people with muscle, bone, or nervous-system injuries or disorders.

Podiatrists specialize in treating feet.

Nutritionists advise patients on dietary concerns.

Orthopedic surgeons diagnose and treat injuries or disorders involving bones, muscles, and joints. They specialize in surgical procedures.

Medical

Drugs

The first step in treating pain is often medication. The complete goal of medical care should focus on reducing inflammation, slowing progress of the disease, preventing permanent joint damage, improving function of a joint through surgery if necessary, and keeping patients functional. Because there is no single treatment that accomplishes all of these goals, a combination of several treatments is usually your best bet. Remember: different people benefit from different combinations.

An analgesic is a painkiller. It does not reduce inflammation. An anti-inflammatory drug reduces redness and swelling.

There is a difference between a side effect and an allergic reaction. Allergies are rare, but if there is a skin rash, wheezing in the lungs, or a runny nose, it is probably an allergic reaction. Nausea, abdominal pain, ringing in the ears, and headache are usually side effects. Allergic reaction means the medication should be avoided in the future. Side effects mean you need a trick to get your body to accept the drug, or perhaps the dosage should be reduced.

Why doesn't science come up with a painkiller for medical and hospital bills?

When should medicine be taken?

Circadian Rhythms

Timing is very important with medications. When you take your medication, the blood and tissue levels rise for a time and then fall as the drug is eliminated from the body. The time until one-half of the drug has been eliminated is called the half-life. This is the time when the effect of the drug begins to wear off and you may need another dose. Different medications have different half-lives. If you want a medication's effect for a certain time—say, midnight, when you want to sleep comfortably—check with your pharmacist for the best time to take it.

———

It's important to know when your body's needs are greatest. Your 24-hour physiological cycle, the circadian rhythm, affects the function of blood pressure, hormone levels, cell growth and division, stomach activity, and other functions which vary predictably during this 24-hour period. Other examples of body cycles, such as the menstrual cycle and allergic reactions, tend to be monthly or seasonal. Understanding these cycles may allow more efficient medicating. More of the drug can be delivered when the disease is more active, and less when the disease is less active.

Currently there are no arthritis medications specifically designed for chronotherapy, the synchronization of medications to the circadian rhythms. This chronotherapy principle can be applied to nonsteroidal anti-inflammatory drugs (NSAIDs). NSAIDs seem to cause more adverse side effects in the morning than in the evening. So, it isn't usually best to take a nighttime NSAID that peaks four to ten hours after taking it. With steroids, prescribed for severe RA, side effects are less if they are taken in the morning so they mimic the natural rhythm of these hormones in the body. The best time to take medication for OA may depend on its release characteristics. A once-a-day or sustained-release preparation that will peak ten to 14 hours later should be taken sometime around noon. Although in one study, when patients with OA took their NSAID at eight a.m., one-third experienced side effects while only seven percent suffered side effects after taking the medication at eight p.m.

———

If you have been told to take medication in the morning, it generally means at the end of your sleep cycle. If you work until seven a.m. and sleep until three p.m., "morning" for you is actually afternoon.

> *NSAIDs seem to cause more adverse side effects in the morning than in the evening.*

> *"The best and most efficient pharmacy is within your own system."*
>
> —Robert Peale, M.D.

The Body's Natural FDA . . .

Food delays absorption of drugs into your body. In some cases it can totally prevent the absorption. Food, though, can also protect the stomach lining and can make taking a drug more comfortable. Antacids perform the same function as do some coatings on medications. The coating is designed to dissolve after the tablet has gone through the stomach and into the small intestine. For some it is helpful. Occasionally, the coating never dissolves and, consequently, no medication is absorbed.

Reinventing the Sandwich . . .

The "sandwich method" can alleviate some gastric problems caused by medications: Eat a little food, take your medications, eat a little more food.

Medical

Drugs and Nutrients—
What Affects What

- **PENICILLAMINE**. This drug may increase your need for vitamin B_6 and zinc.

- **ZINC**. Supplements of this mineral can make drug-induced lupus worse.

- Excess **VITAMIN D**. Too much vitamin D can lead to deposits of calcium on already-damaged joints in patients with gout and rheumatoid arthritis.

- **COLCHICINE**. This gout drug can inhibit your ability to absorb vitamin A and may adversely affect potassium levels.

- **PROBENECID**. Another gout drug, Probenecid decreases the body's absorption of riboflavin (vitamin B_2) and may affect potassium levels.

- **CORTISONE DRUGS**. These drugs, such as Prednisone, interfere with the body's calcium balance and cause you to lose zinc. They may also adversely affect potassium levels.

- **ANTI-INFLAMMATORY DRUGS**. Combined with RA inflammation, these drugs may increase the need for vitamin C.

Drugs are chemicals. If used incorrectly or abused, they can be dangerous.

A Rose is a Rose . . .

According to *Arthritis Today*, a generic drug is essentially a copy of a brand-name drug developed and marketed by another company. FDA standards require the generic drug to have the same active ingredients, dosage breakdowns, strengths, and forms as does the brand-name drug. The generic drug must be bioequivalent to, or act on the body the same way as, the brand-name drug. The root word "equivalent" here does not necessarily mean "equal to." A ten- to 20-percent variation is legally acceptable, although most generics do not vary more than five to six percent. The main difference between generic and brand-name drugs are the fillers and binder. The manufacturer can use any inactive ingredients as long as they don't alter the effectiveness of the active ingredients. For people with allergies, this can be important. You can choose a generic form without the dye if you are allergic to a certain dye in the brand-name drug, or vice-versa.

Generics may not be the best choice for everybody, but they're less expensive. If you choose a generic drug, ask your pharmacist for its rating. Those rated "A" tend to be interchangeable with the brand name. To find the rating of any drug, ask your pharmacist to show you what is known as the "Orange Book," formally titled *Approved Drug Products with Therapeutic Equivalence Evaluations,* which lists the FDA rating of every drug and manufacturer. Stick with "A" drugs.

Generic Aspirin

Aspirin can be found in drugstores under several hundred different formulations. Its effects differ according to which marketing campaign is active. Some forms call themselves "arthritis aspirin," "extra-strength," or "buffered." Basically, they are all just aspirin in various dosages with various additives.

A standard aspirin table is 325 milligrams. It doesn't need a fancy name or to be expensive to work. Additives, such as caffeine or antihistamines, are not necessary and may be contraindicated (specifically advised against for certain people and/or illnesses). Added antacids may be beneficial. However, taking them separately is just as effective and often less expensive.

PHEW!

If aspirin smells like vinegar, it's old. Discard it immediately.

> *Aspirin doesn't need a fancy name or to be expensive to work.*

> *Never store drugs in a humid area or in an excessively hot or excessively cold area.*

Drug Disposal

Flush old medicines down the toilet. Don't throw them in the trash. They can be harmful to children or pets.

––––––––

Adult-Proof Caps?

If you have difficulty with the child-proof caps, ask the pharmacist for a regular top and store the medication someplace inaccessible to children. Never store medications in containers other than their original containers. Separating the label from the medication may cause confusion in dosage and timing instruction as well as in identifying the drug. Every year poisonings occur because people get confused and take the wrong medications or take them incorrectly. Do not trust your memory! Trust the drugstore's labels only! These labels have vital instructions that are specific for you.

––––––––

Drug Storage

Never store drugs in a humid area or in an excessively hot or excessively cold area. Above the stove or beside the shower may not be ideal storage areas.

Medical

1. When should I take it?

2. How long should I take it?

3. Can this drug be taken with other medications?

4. Is there a generic form and can I take it?

5. Are there other less expensive alternatives?

6. What benefits will I notice and how soon will these be apparent?

7. What side effects might I experience and what should I do about them?

8. Can I stop taking the medicine if I feel better? If I feel no effect or feel worse, can I stop on my own or should I consult a physician?

9. When and how will this drug be assessed for benefits and/or toxicity?

10. What should I do if I miss a dose?

11. Under what conditions can I increase or decrease the total daily dose of my medication?

Eleven Questions to Ask Your Pharmacist or Doctor about Your Medications

> **_Let your pharmacy know if a drug is less expensive somewhere else. They may match the price, or in some cases beat it._**

To Reduce Side Effects—

✓ Take medications as prescribed.

✓ Try the "sandwich method." (See page 24.)

✓ Be careful about drinking alcohol.

✓ Monitor yourself and your body's reactions.

———

To Reduce Medication Costs—

1. Ask your doctor about taking the generic form.
2. Ask about switching to a less expensive drug.
3. Take your medication as prescribed. Don't save some of it for later. You may spend more money in the long run because of a relapse.
4. Try to reduce the amount of narcotic pain relievers and tranquilizers. Substitute other forms of pain relief, such as relaxation techniques, hot baths, cold packs, energy conservation, mental distraction, and exercise.
5. Carefully check labels on over-the-counter drugs. Brand-name drugs are often more expensive than generics. Don't pay for ingredients such as caffeine.
6. Shop for the best prices. Let your pharmacy know if a drug is less expensive somewhere else. They may match the price, or in some cases beat it.

Medical

Ten

Medication

Don'ts

1. Don't stop taking your medicine on your own. Seek your doctor's permission first.

2. Don't use someone else's medication or let them use yours.

3. Don't drive or operate heavy machinery if you feel drowsy from medication.

4. Don't mix different medications in one container. Harmful chemical interactions could occur.

5. Don't break medications in half or dilute them in liquid unless this is okayed by your physician or pharmacist.

6. Don't run out of medications. Monitor your supply and plan ahead.

7. Don't take old medications. Dispose of them properly (see page 28).

8. Don't change the dosage on your own. Just because one is good doesn't mean two is better.

9. Don't expect medication alone to do the job.

10. Don't drink alcohol while taking your medications.

32

Drug Strategies:

First-line and

Second-line

Drugs

Doctors usually divide medications into first-line and second-line drugs.

The first-line drugs are usually—not always—tried first and include nonsteroidal anti-inflammatory drugs (NSAIDs). First-line drugs that are used almost exclusively for the treatment of rheumatoid arthritis include steroids, such as Prednisone and Cortisone.

Second-line drugs are used to treat only rheumatoid arthritis and are sometimes called disease-modifying or disease-remittive drugs because there is a correlation between their use and remissions. They include gold salts in the form of shots or pills; Plaquenil, or hydroxy chloroquine, a drug also used to treat malaria; penicillamine, a cousin of the famous antibiotic; and methotrexate and other immunosuppressive drugs that are used to treat cancer.

Medical

NSAIDs (Nonsteroidal Anti-inflammatory Drugs)

First-Line

Drugs

The use of NSAIDs dates back to around 400 B.C. when, legend has it, Hippocrates made a drink from the bark of a willow tree to ease his patients' headaches and labor pains. The main ingredient, a salicylate, is still widely used today and is a subset of NSAIDs. This chemical works fast and blocks the production of prostaglandins, which are accomplices in creating pain and inflammation. Prostaglandins dilate your blood vessels and allow an increased blood flow to sites of injury or infection. They can also cause fever and indirectly promote weakening of the bone and a loss of cartilage. This adds to the tissue destruction in some forms of arthritis.

———

The over-the-counter (OTC) NSAIDs may be used as needed for minor aches and pains and fever reduction. Popular name brands include Anacin, Bayer, Bufferin, Ecotrin, Excedrin, Aleve, Advil, Motrin, and Nuprin. To reduce inflammation, larger doses must be taken than recommended on the bottle. Prescription-strength brands include Voltaren, Dolobid, Ansaid, Indocin, Relafen, Naprosyn, Daypro, Feldene, Clinoril, and Toletin.

All NSAIDs should be taken with food.

Some ulcers are caused by inflammation of the wishbone.

———

The major drawback with salicylates is stomach distress. By inhibiting the stomach's natural defenses, NSAIDs can allow gastric acids to erode the stomach lining, causing internal bleeding and pain. Some types have been developed that do not dissolve until they reach the small intestine. Other forms include time-released tablets and capsules that allow medication to enter the bloodstream slowly and, hopefully, reduce stomach irritation. Some types have even been chemically modified to be easier on the stomach. Medications such as Tagamet, Zantac, and Prilosec are sometimes prescribed in conjunction with NSAIDs to prevent ulcer formation.

———

Nonacetylated salicylates is a group of NSAIDs that are similar to aspirin but chemically modified to be easier on the stomach. They include such medications as choline magnesium trisalicylate (Trilisate) and salsalate (Disalcid). Ask your doctor for more information.

To avoid toxicity, consult the *Physician's Desk Reference* regarding the percentage of people who develop toxicities for the drug you are taking.

———

Be an avid label reader. Don't over-medicate yourself. Toxicity can sometimes occur when over-the-counter drugs you take for unrelated problems, such as stomach upset or colds, contain an ingredient that you are already taking. For example, if you are taking Ansaid and then drink Alka-Seltzer, you may be getting too much aspirin.

———

Another reason toxicity occurs is that many of the newer potent anti-inflammatory drugs, such as Feldene, are only available in fixed dosages. That means a 100-pound woman would take the same amount of a drug as a 240-pound fullback. Guess who suffers the most side effects. To avoid damage to your kidneys and liver, get regular urine and blood tests that can detect damage. Educate yourself about the fixed dosages. If you are a 100-pound woman and the drug you're taking comes only in a fixed dosage, ask your doctor about cutting the pills in half.

> *High doses of corticosteroids are limited to short-term use during flares.*

Corticosteroids

When corticosteroids were developed over 50 years ago, people thought the cure for arthritis had been found. Time has an uncanny way of throwing curve balls, however, and they turned out not to be the answer. The curve was their undesirable side effects after high doses were given long term. Now high doses are limited to short-term use during flares and sometimes prescribed as a temporary measure until other drugs can take effect. They are closely related to cortisol, a hormone naturally produced in the outer layer (cortex) of your adrenal glands, one of which sits on top of each of your kidneys. (Commit that to memory. It may come in handy during your next parlor game!) They are very different from the sex steroids, or androgens, taken by athletes which have no role in treating arthritis. Cortisol helps regulate salt and water balance, and carbohydrate, fat, and protein metabolism. It's released in increased amounts during times of stress or injury, and can produce a feeling of well-being, sometimes even exhilaration.

———

The birth of corticosteroids emanated from the birth process itself. Scientists noticed that women with rheumatoid arthritis improved during pregnancy. Researchers investigated what chemical changes might be responsible.

Medical

Corticosteroids—Wisely Used

Corticosteroids can be taken orally or intravenously for broad systemic effects. When just a few joints are affected by arthritis, occasionally injecting a corticosteroid compound directly into those joints may provide temporary relief. Familiar names include Prednisone, Cortisone, Decadron, Medrol, Pediapred, Deltasone, Aristocort, and Hydrocortone.

———

They should be taken with food and should not be stopped abruptly. Sudden suspension or interruption can lead to an adrenal crisis. The dosage must be tapered or reduced gradually to allow your own adrenal glands to return to normal function.

———

Side effects include weight gain, thin skin, muscle weakness, brittle bones, increased appetite, indigestion, acne, cataracts, diabetes, insomnia, mood changes, and restlessness. They can also reduce resistance to, and mask symptoms of, infection.

Anyone taking corticosteroids should wear a medic alert bracelet.

> *Money may well be the best analgesic.*

Analgesics

Analgesic is a fancy word for pain reliever. An analgesic does not inhibit prostaglandin production and is therefore not effective for treating inflammation. It acts by blocking pain perception and reducing fever.

———

Common over-the-counter brands include Tylenol, Bayer Select, Panadol, Excedrin, Anacin, and Percogesic. Narcotic analgesics include Fioricet and Phenaphen with codeine, Tylenol with codeine, Percodan, Darvon, PC-Cap, and Wygesic. Narcotic analgesics require a prescription.

———

Because the narcotic analgesics do not have FDA-approved indications for arthritis and because they may cause psychological and physical dependence, some doctors feel they should only be used to treat severe flares and for the short term. A trend has begun, however, where many professionals believe the relief offered by these medications outweigh the slight risk of addiction. Use caution with narcotic analgesics if you have a history of alcohol abuse, kidney disease, hepatitis, depression, or liver disease.

Medical

Slow Gold

With SAARDs (slow-acting antirheumatic drugs) also called "DMARDs" (disease-modifying, anti-rheumatic drugs), patience is a must. These drugs aren't called slow-acting for nothing. Gold treatments may take months before the improvements are noticed.

———

The drugs in this group are used primarily to treat rheumatoid arthritis, although some are prescribed for lupus, ankylosing spondylitis and Sjögren's syndrome. They are often called the second line of defense and are used only when other less-potent drugs fail.

———

These drugs go by a variety of names, including remittive and slow-acting, which tell you something about the way in which they work. Remittive means they may slow down the disease process, though that only occasionally results in complete remission. Slow-acting means just that— it acts slowly. Sometimes it may take six to eight months for the slow-acting drug to produce a response.

> *Instructions can range from "take on an empty stomach" to "take with food."*

SAARDs or DMARDs work by reducing some of the signs of inflammation—although they aren't generally anti-inflammatory—and preventing or retarding joint erosion. They do not reduce prostaglandin production or relieve pain, but they appear to affect the body's immune system in helpful ways. The exact workings of the drugs are not fully understood yet. If your arthritis is troublesome, but not causing progressive joint damage, the risk of side effects may outweigh the potential benefits.

———

Included in this category are gold treatments, both oral and intravenous (Ridaura); hydroxy chloroquine (Plaquenil); penicillamine (Cuprimine, Depen); methotrexate (Rheumatrex); and sulfasalazine (Azulfidine).

———

Their side effects can range from rashes and diarrhea, to vision impairment.

———

Special instructions can range from "take on an empty stomach" to "take with food." Each drug is very different so it is important to follow the doctor's and/or the pharmacist's directions.

Medical

Bone-Building Medications

Bone-building medications help restore the balance between the normal breakdown of the bones and their rebuilding. Age, loss of estrogen, or corticosteroid use are frequent inhibitors of the building process.

———

Recognized brand names include Calcimar, Niacalcin, Premarin, PMB, and Didronel. Their effect may not be evident immediately, but eventually they should reduce the occurrence of fractures if that has been a problem in the past.

———

Tranquilizers

Tranquilizers and muscle relaxants also may be prescribed to reduce muscle tension and spasms. Like narcotic pain relievers, these drugs may be addictive and should only be used for short periods of time.

Their effect may not be evident immediately, but eventually they should reduce the occurrence of fractures if that has been a problem in the past.

> **They seem to allow the sufferers to get the deep restorative sleep they lack.**

Tricyclic Antidepressants

The main usage of tricyclic antidepressants for arthritis sufferers is to treat fibromyalgia—a common arthritis-related condition. The antidepressants seem to allow the sufferers to get the deep restorative sleep they lack, which consequently aids pain relief and provides increased energy.

———

Dosage amounts are usually less than those given to relieve pain.

———

Common names are Elavil, Endep, Triavil, Norpramin, Adapin, Sinequan, Tipramine, Tofranil, Pamelor, and Surmontil.

———

Their side effects range from weight gain, dizziness, and headaches, to dry mouth and drowsiness.

Medical

Despite gout's shady reputation (it has often been associated with wine imbibing and throbbing big toes—enough said), it's a torturous disease. In gout, excess uric acid in the blood turns to crystals that deposit in the joints.

———

The first step is pain relief. Colchicine, which is often immediately prescribed, reduces the inflammation within hours. The next step is preventing future attacks. A maintenance prescription of allopurinol may be preventative if an overproduction of uric acid is at the root. If the excess uric acid in the blood is caused by an inability to excrete uric acid, a maintenance prescription of Probenecid may be given. The success rate of these drugs is encouraging though the initial results may be discouraging—increased rate of attacks as the body responds to the drug and tries to normalize.

———

Common brand names: Lopurin, Zyloprim, Colchicine, Benemid, and Probalan. Take on an empty stomach. Side effects can include hives, skin rashes, diarrhea, and headache.

———

One therapy alternative is adrenocorticotrophic hormone (ACTH), a synthetic version of a hormone that helps control the body's secretion of inflammation-controlling corticosteroids. It seems to work faster than NSAIDs.

The best medicine for rheumatism is being thankful it isn't gout!

> *The most common results of surgery are success and satisfaction.*

Under the Knife . . .

Although most arthritis patients won't need surgery, for some it's an option that improves their lifestyle. Often the main reason for surgery is pain relief. It may also produce an increased ability to use joints. Surgery is also done to correct deformities, which can result in cosmetic improvement as well as heightened usefulness, especially when the hands are involved.

———

The most common results of surgery are success and satisfaction. And this is not always the case. Sometimes a joint is worse after surgery. Recovery periods can also be lengthy. Add to that the other risks associated with surgery as well as the expense, and you realize that you have a very serious decision to make. That is why it is important to research your options carefully.

Medical

Now, Later, or Never . . .

Surgical procedures keep improving with time. That is why the longer you wait, the more advanced the surgical technique will be. It's the same with replacement joints. The joints have a limited life span, so the longer you can wait the better. Be sure to allow enough time to get several opinions. Don't make hasty decisions. Find the leading surgeon in your area. Investigate the success rates of this procedure. Talk to people who have undergone this particular surgery.

———

This does not mean, however, that it is always best to wait. Some conditions, such as tendon rupture, bone or joint infections, can require surgery immediately.

———

The most likely candidates for surgery are those with severe and debilitating osteoarthritis and rheumatoid arthritis. Joint surgery is not usually performed for people with lupus, scleroderma, or gout.

> *The longer you wait, the more advanced the surgical technique will be.*

Before taking

the plunge . . .

If surgery seems imminent, discuss with the proper medical personnel—

- ✓ various risks
- ✓ anticipated pain relief
- ✓ quality-of-life improvement
- ✓ projected recovery time
- ✓ possible rehabilitation programs
- ✓ possible complications

Ask yourself—

- ✓ Is my pain unacceptable?
- ✓ Am I requiring narcotic pain relievers?
- ✓ Have I exhausted all other pain-relief options?
- ✓ Do I have realistic goals and expectations?
- ✓ How healthy am I overall?

———

Some doctors recommend an orthopedic consultation when 1) the patient has failed to respond to physical pain-relief methods and drug therapy and 2) the pain is unrelenting and disabling. When OA patients are in severe pain, it has been found that no drug will really provide relief. Surgery can, though!

Medical

U.S. News and World Report and the National Opinion Research Center conduct an annual survey of 2,400 physicians in 16 medical specialties. In 1997, the doctors nominated the five hospitals they considered best for their specialty from among 1,631 major academic institutions and specialized medical centers, ignoring location and expense. The results are obviously subjective and in no way imply that other institutions are less effective.

1. Mayo Clinic
Rochester, MN 55905
(507) 284-2511

2. Hospital for Special Surgery
New York, NY 10021
(212) 606-1000

3. Mass. General Hospital
Boston, MA 02114
(617)726-2000

4. Johns Hopkins Hospital
Baltimore, MD 21287
(410)955-5464

5. Duke Univ. Medical Center
Durham, NC 27710
(919) 684-8111

6. UCLA Medical Center
Los Angeles, CA 90095
(310) 825-9111

7. Cleveland Clinic Foundation
Cleveland, OH 44195
(216) 444-2200

8. Hospital for Joint Diseases
New York, NY 10003
(212) 598-6000

9. Univ. of Washington
Medical Center
Seattle, WA
(206) 548-3300

10. Univ. of Iowa Hospitals
Iowa City, IA 52242
(319) 356-1616

Synovectomy:

This can buy

time.

The most frequently performed surgeries are—

Synovectomy—cutting out of the synovial membrane.
Osteotomy—cutting out bone to allow improved alignment.
Resection—cutting out all or part of a bone to relieve pain.
Arthroplasty—joint reconstruction.

Synovectomy

A synovectomy is the cutting out of the synovial membrane, or the synovium. The synovium is the cells lining the joint capsule, which secrete lubricating fluid. Removing the grossly inflamed synovial lining of the joint can be performed through a surgical incision or an arthroscope depending on the size of the joint. The joint is opened and tissues and other components are removed, leaving enough synovium to maintain lubrication.

Recovery may take several weeks. Rehabilitation is gradual and includes range-of-motion and strengthening exercises. Often cure isn't permanent. Over time the synovium grows back. Synovectomy is performed on a host of joints including shoulders, elbows, hips, and knees, and on the tendons on the back of the hand to prevent additional tears. It provides good pain relief and is more conservative than joint replacement.

Osteotomy

An osteotomy is surgically removing the bone to allow realignment in a better position. The bone is cut or remodeled so that weight is more evenly distributed. In corrective surgery of the knee, a piece of bone may be removed from one of the leg bones to allow better alignment.

———

Osteotomies afford good pain relief (70 percent to 85 percent initially) but deterioration does occur over time. This procedure is recommended for younger patients. Recovery may take several weeks.

———

Resection

Resection is the surgical removal of all or part of a damaged bone to relieve pain. Resection is indicated when affected bones become too painful. This type of procedure is also used to remove bunions.

Osteotomies afford good pain relief.

Arthroplasty:

This is by far the most important orthopedic surgical procedure for arthritis.

Arthroplasty

Arthroplasty involves joint reconstruction using the patient's own tissues as well as artificial joint components. Most arthroplasties involve a total joint replacement with a man-made prosthesis.

———

This is by far the most important orthopedic surgical procedure for arthritis. Several hundred thousand joint-replacement operations are performed annually in the United States. Total hip replacements are the most successful surgery in this category, followed by knee and knuckle replacement. Ankle and shoulder replacements are performed less frequently. These surgeries are over 90-percent effective in relieving pain and in significantly restoring function to the joint. Operations to replace the small joints of the fingers are widely practiced, but the outcomes haven't been generally satisfactory.

———

The joint is removed and replaced with an artificial one. The cartilage is replaced by a long-wearing plastic, the bone is replaced by stainless steel, and the artificial joint is embedded in the ends of the bones on either side by an effective cement, methyl methacrylate.

———

Recovery times vary from six weeks to several months.

Total hip replacements have been performed for over 25 years and, in a 20-year follow-up study, fifty percent of the patients in one study performed at least light labor, including maintaining a home, performing house cleaning, and mowing the lawn.

The present artificial hip is estimated to last 10 to 15 years. Newer models are expected to last longer.

Recent studies demonstrate the cost effectiveness of total hip replacement. Compared with both surgical treatment of coronary artery disease and medical treatment of hypertension, hip replacement is a more effective medical intervention, using quality-adjusted years as an endpoint.

Arthroplasty:

Total Hip

Replacement

Arthrodesis
fuses a joint to
relieve pain or
give support.

Arthrodesis (Fusion)

Arthrodesis fuses a joint to relieve pain or give support. It involves the fusing together of bones into a fixed position.

———

The bones are surgically repositioned into the best, most functional alignment possible. The fusion provides a platform for movement and prevents pain in the fused area. The joint can no longer bend in its usual way, however, and natural motion is lost.

———

This procedure may be considered for patients whose bones are not healthy enough for a joint-replacement operation, for those who have repeated joint infections that do not allow the insertion of a prosthesis, and for small joints like the thumb, where joint replacements are done less frequently.

———

Recovery can take several months and braces may need to be worn. The fusions do not always work and nonunion can occur.

Medical

A survey of 1,051 patients who had joint surgery offered these bits of advice—

✓ Have it done!

✓ Think it through.

✓ Get several opinions.

✓ Choose your surgeon carefully.

✓ Consider donating your own blood weeks prior to the surgery.

✓ Pick the best hospital available.

✓ Learn everything you can about the procedure beforehand.

✓ Get in shape.

✓ Prepare your family for the role they will play.

✓ Follow post-op instructions.

✓ Be realistic.

✓ Think positively.

"Oh, my friend, it's not what they take away from you that counts. It's what you do with what you have left."

—Hubert Humphrey after cancer surgery

Folks for whom surgery is not the best choice:

✓ People who are bedridden.

✓ People who spend most of their time in a wheel chair.

✓ People with advanced cardiovascular or renal disease.

✓ People unwilling to undergo proper rehab.

✓ People who have severe arthritis in other limbs that prevent the use of crutches or canes.

Medical

Many of tomorrow's best treatments may not be in the discovery of new drugs, but in using old drugs in new ways. By combining methotrexate, a second-line drug prescribed for RA, and cyclosporin, a drug developed to prevent rejection of transplanted organs, researchers found the patients had fewer tender and swollen joints and noted significantly less pain than patients taking methotrexate alone.

———

While drug therapy is often the first treatment prescribed by a doctor to reduce pain, it is almost never the only therapy. Many others exist and, again, trial and error is often the only way to figure out what works for you.

New Arthritis

Treatment

Ideas . . .

> *"All the scholastic scaffolding falls, as a ruined edifice, before a single word: faith."*
>
> — Napoleon Bonaparte

Through the Skin

Some anti-inflammatory drugs might be more effective if delivered directly to the joints through the skin. The problem has been developing a drug "escort" to get them through (The skin is an excellent guardian barrier.) without irritation and inflammation. Dr. J. Howard Rytting of the Department of Pharmaceutical Chemistry at the University of Kansas at Lawrence reported that he and his colleagues may have found the solution. The secret is that their escorts are biodegradable. This method of drug administration will be best used for fairly potent, low-dose drugs, particularly when oral administration has some drawback.

―――――

Lupus Measurement

Standard lab tests do not always give accurate indications of lupus' progress. To remedy this problem, several newer ways of measuring lupus activity have been developed. The new tests seem to indicate the overall state of the disease and the patient more thoroughly than simple laboratory tests.

Medical

Injectable Bone

Doctors at three U.S. medical centers found promising results from a toothpaste-like mixture of calcium phosphate compounds and a sodium phosphate solution. This can be injected directly into a fracture site to hold bone fragments in place. Tests found the compound to be virtually identical to natural bone.

Bones and Depression

In a study published in the American Journal of Psychiatry, doctors found that people who were severely depressed—and thus had produced higher levels of cortisol—were more likely to have osteoporosis than those who weren't. This study has identified depression as a clinical risk for developing osteoporosis.

Vaccinations

Some doctors believe repeated vaccinations of properly prepared forming cells will sufficiently curb the immune reaction to hinder arthritic inflammation. Other researchers are genetically engineering cells to inject directly into knuckles, where the injected cells can teach the immune system to stop attacking the body's own cartilage.

New arthritis

treatment

ideas . . .

> *Until recently, there has been no procedure to reveal the subtle changes in tissue that occur in the early stages of the arthritis.*

Watching Arthritis

Regular x-rays aren't specific enough to see the subtle changes in tissue of early arthritis. Martha Gray, an MIT professor of electrical engineering and the interim director of the Harvard-MIT Division of Health Sciences and Technology, is helping to develop a technique which will allow "watching the disease happen." The technique may finally provide a reliable way to test drug efficacy by measuring concentrations of an important component of cartilage, proteoglycan.

New NSAIDs

New NSAIDs are being developed that release nitric oxide. This stimulates blood flow and healing in the stomach. According to the national medical spokesperson for the Arthritis Society, such new drugs look very promising.

Arthritis Suppression

Genetic engineers have piggybacked a gene capable of blocking interleukin-1, a key component in the body's immune system, onto a harmless virus. This altered virus suppressed arthritis in rabbits. The treatment is still in the experimental stage and needs further refinement.

Medical

Two New Drugs

Two new arthritis drugs should become available in 1997. The first may be a combination of the NSAID diclofenac and the cytoprotective agent misoprostol (Arthrotec). The combination may reduce peptic ulcers by up to 50 percent. The other, tenidap (Enable), is a novel agent that interferes with cytokines, thus blocking pain and inflammation. This drug will probably be more useful in patients with rheumatoid arthritis.

———

Cultured Cartilage

Laboratory-cultured cartilage is being researched as a possibility to combat the effects of osteoarthritis. At present, orthopedic surgeons replace roughly 600,000 knees, hips, and shoulders each year in the United States. Chondrocytes removed from an individual could be grown in an artificial matrix until they generate healthy connective tissue that could be implanted on the surface of a worn-down joint.

More new

arthritis

treatment

ideas . . .

Something

smells

fishy here!

The verdict is still out on the exact role that fish oil may play in arthritis treatment. "It does appear that fish oil provides an alternative building block for molecules that participate in the inflammatory process," says Dr. John Krehmer, head of Rheumatology at Albany Medical College. The end products formed from fish oils have beneficial effects on dampening inflammation and perhaps some elements of the immune response associated with the disease.

———

Fish oil may also affect the way cells in the body signal each other. Experts do caution that the results from using fish oil are modest, and some people object to the taste, cost, and stomach distress it can cause.

———

Fish-oil capsules should be taken under a doctor's supervision. Adding salmon, tuna, mackerel, or herring to your diet is a way to naturally add fish oil, and it's healthy (unless you're the fish).

Forget the remedy that claims to cure or fix a lot of diseases! There are no universal treatments. Be suspicious of so-called "secret" remedies.

———

These remedies have been tested scientifically: seaweed, immune milk, snake venom, red-ant serum, Certo, honey and vinegar, alfalfa, and special arthritis diets. Valid scientific studies have not proven that such remedies work.

———

Nitroimidazoles are antibiotics for amoebic infections Studies to see if they help RA show they're a little more helpful than standard drugs, but have many more side effects.

———

Laser treatment: One controlled study did not show any benefit when compared with placebo laser treatment. But laser technology is in its infancy. It may yet prove useful.

———

Cod-liver oil can be dangerous. It contains large doses of vitamins A and D, which can be toxic. The idea of oil taken by mouth lubricating the joints is unsound. Oils are broken down before absorption into the bloodstream.

———

Vitamins, zinc and copper: No valid studies support their value. Doses recommended anecdotally as "therapeutic" may cause significant side effects.

Tube therapy:

While rub-on balms and creams are rarely ever prescribed by doctors, many people swear they are beneficial. Even though there is little scientific evidence to support their use, *Arthritis Today* devoted a section of their drug guide to "pain relief in a tube." Thus, the therapeutic benefit seems widely acknowledged. The Arthritis Foundation includes "topical creams" in its list of "harmless baloney" along with copper bracelets in "Arthritis—Unproven Remedies." Just remember: If it works, use it!

Also called topical analgesics (pain relievers), these preparations are often counterirritants. That is, they make you forget about pain by irritating your skin to make it feel hot. The heat in turn may soothe some soreness and stiffness. They work by stimulating the nerve endings which distract the brain's attention from the greater source of discomfort.

The irritating ingredients may be menthol, oil of wintergreen, camphor, eucalyptus oil, turpentine oil, dihydrochloride, or methylnicotinate. Topical non-prescription creams containing capsaicin may be combined with other medications to temporarily relieve pain by decreasing a neurotransmitter called substance P.

Medical

Salicylate is another ingredient often found in the compounds. It decreases the ability of the nerve ending in the skin to sense pain. Some studies suggest that they also work through skin absorption.

————

Even though these drugs come in creams, salves, or gels, and their brand names are almost household words, they are still potent chemicals which require caution. If you are allergic to aspirin, you should check with your doctor before using an ointment with salicylates. Products which contain capsaicin may not be appropriate if you have diabetic neuropathy. Become a label reader if you aren't one now and never hesitate to ask questions.

————

Topical creams should not be applied before external heating devices are used. They can cause burns.

Familiar and widely used, these ointments are still potent chemicals which require caution.

From the Notebook of You've-Got-To-Be-Kidding Remedies:

✓ Sitting in a uranium mine for two hours a day

✓ Copper bracelets

✓ Seaweed bracelets

✓ WD-40 sprayed on the joints

✓ Vibrating chairs and beds

✓ Injections of turtle blood

✓ Mussel extract

✓ Covering your body with cow manure twice a day

Medical

ASK!

✓ Is this research associated with a medical facility?

✓ Is there a scientific reason to think the results are reliable?

✓ Were the people in the study like you—the same age, sex and type of arthritis?

✓ Has the research been published in a medical journal?

✓ Does the report suggest health actions that people should take as a result of the research?

Where to Go for Help

The Arthritis Foundation is unparalleled in its assistance to arthritis sufferers. Call (800) 283-7800 for your local chapter and area services.

Research—How to know if it is valid.

Ouch! It Hurts!

Unfortunately, pain is a byproduct of arthritis. You can become a better pain manager by understanding some important aspects of pain.

———

Acute means sudden, intense and severe. Chronic means incurable, long lasting, and continuing. Whether you experience one or both types of pain may depend on your type of arthritis. In either case, pain isn't fun. Some say arthritis pain is like a mother-in-law's visit: "It was a surprise, the duration was a mystery, and the presence constant and grating."

———

Pain is not simply a matter of nerves and neurotransmitters, a sensation passing from the site of tissue damage to the brain," says David Morris, author of *The Culture of Pain*. When a pain signal reaches the brain, it meshes with remembered experience and thus becomes unique to that moment in a person's life. What you think and feel can dramatically affect the pain you experience, including the intensity and your endurance. This does not mean "it's all in your head." Quite the contrary. Pain is always real to the person who experiences it. There is pain with no known cause and with no observable damage, and there is no imaginary pain.

Pain Management

Normally pain is the body's alarm system. It tells you in no uncertain terms, "We've got a problem." Because of its intensity, you listen. You take appropriate measures to alleviate the pain, like removing your hand from the hot stove. With arthritis, however, it is not as simple. Yes, the realization that something is wrong is loud and clear, but relieving it is not as easy. To make matters more complicated, what works for some may not work for others.

With arthritis, the pain is often caused by inflammation, joint tissue damage, muscle strain, and/or fatigue. Along with the resultant physical changes such as movement limitations, the emotional ups and downs can add to the pain and trap you in a cycle that is hard to break. Increased disease activity, stress, excessive physical activity, dwelling on pain, fatigue, anxiety, and depression can make pain feel worse.

Dwelling on pain, fatigue, anxiety, and depression can make pain feel worse.

In a word . . .

Before a doctor can fully understand the extent of your pain, you must clearly and accurately express what and how you feel. "It just hurts," isn't very specific. By using descriptive words your physician will be better able to treat you. Below is a list of words that may be helpful to you or go pull out your handy thesaurus.

Painful Adjectives

wrenching HOT SEARING tingling STINGING

dull sore tender rasping sickening suffocating

terrifying CRUEL wretched BLINDING annoying

troublesome FLICKERING quivering beating

pounding shooting FLASHING pricking stabbing

sharp gnawing cramping crushing TUGGING

intense spreading radiating piercing tight numb

cool COLD nagging NAUSEATING agonizing

torturing DREADFUL

Pain Management

Who: Everyone, but especially arthritis sufferers, should do all that they can to protect their joints.

Why: Reduce pain, reduce inflammation, preserve joints, stay active

When: Every day, all day

Where: Everywhere

Here we go—

Joint

Protection

Hit List

Joint protection— Here's how!

Respect pain. If pain from an activity lasts more than an hour, or it occurs suddenly and is severe, consider this a warning sign. Try performing the activity differently or limit it altogether. Example: If carrying grocery bags with your hands is painful, carry them next to your body using the arm and shoulder instead. Or, better yet, have someone else carry them for you.

Avoid incorrect postures and positions. They lead to fatigue, pain, strains, and possible deformities. Example: Adjust the height of your computer keyboard to eliminate strain on the wrist and hands. Wear braces or splints if necessary to "train" the joints.

Avoid staying in one position for a long time. Take frequent breaks or stretches every 30 minutes. Example: Get up from your desk for a drink of water at the water fountain at least twice an hour. It will hydrate you and will relieve stiffness.

Use the strongest and largest joints when possible. Direct pressure on the smallest, weakest joints creates undue stress and pain. Remember that fingers are not for bearing weight. Example: Use the palms, not fingers, when pushing up from a chair. Use your body weight to move objects. Example: Close a drawer with your rear end; move a chair with your hips.

Pain Management

Distribute weight to the larger joints. Avoid using the smaller joints, like the hands.

Example: Use shoulder bags or back packs instead of handbags. Carry packages in the arms close to the body instead of using the handles.

Plan ahead for activities that cannot be stopped. Example: If walking a long distance, know where the benches are located so you may stop and rest.

Use labor-saving devices. Example: Invest in electric scissors.

Avoid activities involving tight grasp. Tight grasps happen when you carry heavy objects such as handbags, shopping bags, pails, and baskets by the handles. They also happen when you use screwdrivers, shears, and pliers. Learn to hold everything no tighter than necessary. Tight grasps contribute to ulnar deviation (the shifting of fingers toward the little finger side of the hand) and dislocation of other joints.

More

joint

protection —

Still protecting those joints!

Avoid ulnar pressure on the fingers. Ulnar pressure moves your fingers away from your thumb. Watch your fingers when you do a familiar task. You'll see that the fingers are pushing against each other toward the small finger rather than supporting each other in good alignment. Your joints are more stable in this position and you get more power per pull. Example—Hold a knife like an ice pick and use a pulling action to cut.

Avoid all pressure against the back of your fingers.

Use each joint in its best position.

Keep moving! Follow therapeutic exercise guidelines to increase mobility and strength.

Avoid excessive and constant pressure against the pad of your thumb. This occurs when you pinch too hard. Examples: Opening a car door, sewing through tough fabric.

Pain Management

Balance rest with activity. A person needs at least eight hours of sleep at night and a one-hour rest period during the middle of the afternoon to give their joints adequate time to recover.

Pace yourself. Don't overdo it. Combine a heavy chore with a light one or punctuate each with a short rest. After raking leaves, sit and return phone calls.

Plan ahead. Be organized. Know what you want to accomplish, what you will need to get the job done, and the most efficient way to do it. Example: Take a list with you when marketing. Go down only the aisles that contain the needed items. This eliminates excessive walking.

Prioritize. Do the most important tasks first. If time and energy allow, complete the list. If not, congratulate yourself on accomplishing the main things.

Fatigue Management Hit List

> *Walking fast takes 1 ½ times more energy than walking slowly.*

Allow enough time. That way you do not have to rush at the last minute.

———

Work relaxed. Think pleasant thoughts. Work to classical or soothing music.

———

Adopt a moderate pace. Walking fast takes 1 ½ times more energy than walking slowly. Walking down stairs takes twice as much energy as walking on level ground. Walking up stairs takes seven times as much energy as walking on level ground.

———

Slide objects. Do not lift them, and sit whenever possible.

———

Smile three times more than you frown! Seek pleasant diversions. Watch a bird from the window.

———

Ask for help! Don't be ashamed. Perhaps you could swap shopping with a neighbor. Volunteer to tutor a teenager if they will vacuum for you.

Pain Management

And They're Off . . .

✓ When **walking**, take the same size step with each foot. Bend your knee when moving ahead. Keep it straight when standing on it. Your heel should touch the ground with each step.

✓ Maintain **GOOD POSTURE**. Hold yourself erect but relaxed. Visualize a string coming up from the top of your head and holding you straight.

✓ **Proper support** is the goal. Avoid wearing slippers, high-heels, or thin-soled shoes for long periods. They don't cushion joints. Athletic shoes are "in" for casual and everyday activities. They are lightweight and supportive. Replace regular laces with elastic ones, which convert shoes into slip-ons. The Rockport Company has fashionable shoes, accepted by the American Podiatric Medical Association.

✓ The **Best Time** to buy shoes is mid-afternoon. Look for a steel or rigid shank in the heel; flexibility at the ball of the foot; a broad, high toe box; and laces.

It does not matter how slowly you go as long as you get there.

> *The more eyelets the shoe has, the easier the shoe is to adjust for a custom fit.*

✓ **Buckle** straps can be changed to *hook-and-loop tape* or to a **zipper** at a shoe repair shop. Boots with full-length zippers are easier to manage than pull-ons.

✓ To aid **shoe removal**, there are expanding devices that allow shoe removal without bending.

✓ Shoes with laces need to be **properly laced** for maximum support. The American Orthopedic Foot and Ankle Society recommends that you begin at the bottom of the shoe and tighten the laces one set of eyelets at a time. This prevents unnecessary stress on the top eyelets and provides for a more comfortable shoe fit. The more eyelets the shoe has, the easier the shoe is to adjust for a custom fit.

Pain Management

✓ For **w i d e feet** try buying shoes with staggered eyelets, then lace the ones closest to the tongue of the shoe. The eyelets that are closer together will provide more width.

✓ If you have *sensitive* areas caused by nerve injury, tendon injury, or other causes, simply skip the eyelets at the point of pain.

✓ For **hammer toes**, corns, bleeding toes, or toenail problems, lace shoes so the toe-box area is lifted. To do this start the lacing straight across the bottom then take the left lace and bring it up through the top right eyelet. Then lace the right lace in straight lines from eyelet to eyelet up to the top left eyelet. The toe-box can be adjusted by pulling on the lace that travels directly from the toe to the top of the shoe.

✓ **Custom-made shoes** are an option for people with severe problems. Consult your physician or therapist.

Custom-made shoes are an option for people with severe problems.

> *Canes are usually recommended when only one or two joints on the same side are involved.*

A simple aid, such as a *cane*, may be the best way to stay mobile. Resist the temptation to self-prescribe and self-teach because proper fitting and instruction for use of these devices are vital for their effectiveness. Improper usage can cause more harm than benefit. As always, consult your physician. Canes are usually recommended when only one or two joints on the same side are involved.

The elbow should be almost straight when leaning on the cane and an adjustable metal one is preferable over the static wooden kind. If crutches are advised, remember both hands will be involved so a backpack is a good alternative to a handbag.

Always prop the canes or crutches where they will not fall and can be easily accessed. Attaching a rubber tip to the hooked end of a cane can help keep it in place when hooked over a table edge or shelf. This seems to be common sense, and trying to retrieve fallen aids can be very frustrating.

Pain Management

Chairs should be easy to get into and out of, the right height, and comfortable. Armrests are preferable.

———

Your feet should rest flat on the floor. If this isn't possible use a stool, box, or other object. Keep the knees higher than the hips.

———

The full length of your thighs should rest comfortably on the seat of the chair. Keep your shoulders relaxed.

———

Use a swivel chair to eliminate much twisting and straining when you work at a desk.

———

If you use a pillow for lumbar support, be sure it increases your comfort, not your stiffness and pain. A clutch purse can be substituted for a lumbar pillow if you are out for the evening and find yourself sitting for an extended period.

———

Rise from a chair by sliding forward, placing your feet a few inches apart, and behind your knees. Place your palms (not knuckles) on the arm rests and push down with your hands and legs, bending your head and upper body forward over your knees. Straighten your knees and back until you are erect. Avoid low chairs, rocking chairs, or free-moving chairs.

Taking a load off...

| Sleeping |
| Beautifully |

Sleeping

Beautifully

The correct resting position can do much to reduce fatigue and stiffness. The one-third of your life spent sleeping should be on a firm mattress with proper support. Your body should not sag in the middle of the bed. Place a bed board (use ¾-inch plywood) between the mattress and the box spring to increase firmness.

———

The best position is to sleep on your side or back if your knees or hips are not affected by arthritis. In either case, a small soft pillow to support your neck is advised. Never stack pillows beneath your head. This misaligns the curvature of the neck. Pillows can be used between the knees to relieve back pain. If the hips or knees are affected, your best sleeping position is one where your knees are straight and the hips are in a neutral position, not rotated to the side.

———

To prevent flexion contractures of the hip, try to rest on your stomach for 10 to 15 minutes a day. Put a small pillow under your ankles while you're asleep to keep your knees straight. Never sleep with pillows under your knees even if this is more comfortable. Check with your doctor to see which is best for you.

Pain Management

Pressure redistribution is the answer for some. Foam waffle pads, or electrical pads that alternately inflate and deflate are options. The idea of the devices is to redistribute pressure, retain heat, and dissipate moisture. Check your local department or discount store.

———

Some people use heat during sleep for relief and relaxation. Sources range from a heated water bed to an electric blanket. Sleeping in gloves or snug, heat-retaining socks can provide similar relief without as much expense.

"Always do one thing less than you think you can do."

Bernard Baruch

277 Things

If insomnia is a problem, try these techniques:

✓ Maintain a regular sleep schedule.

✓ Try time-released aspirin to maintain pain relief throughout the night.

✓ Use relaxation techniques to ease body tensions.

✓ Wait until you are very, very, very sleepy (not just a little sleepy) to go to bed.

✗ Avoid caffeine.

✗ Avoid alcohol for three to four hours before bedtime.

✓ Create a comfortable environment.

✓ Take a warm bath.

✗ Avoid exercising immediately before bed.

✗ Do not nap during the day.

✓ Develop a nighttime ritual and stick to it.

Pain Management

The treatment of arthritis often involves reducing pain. There are many ways to treat arthritis and its pain.

Non-medical treatments such as exercise, rest, and applications of heat and cold are included in the remainder of this section.

Diet issues are in the final section on eating for wellness.

Information about pain itself as well as medical treatments, such as drugs and surgery, are covered in the medical chapter.

Pain Relief—
Non-Medical

277 Things

Pain-Relief Remedies and Frequency of Use

Medication	71%
Application of heat	64%
Exercise	63%
Rest	62%
Applying warm water	56%
Applying cold	12%
Ointments and creams	8%
Other	6%
Paraffin baths	4%
Nothing	2%

Pain Management

Relief in Sight

The body naturally creates painkilling substances called endorphins in response to different kinds of controls. These include natural controls, such as your own thoughts and emotions. For example, imagine that a mother who is driving with her child is hurt in a car accident. The mother is so worried about the child that she doesn't feel the pain from her own broken arm. The concern for the child has blocked the pain signal and kept the pain from affecting her. Medicines are also a type of control known as "outside control." Morphine is an example. Exercise, relaxation, massage, heat and cold treatments can also stimulate endorphins or block pain signals. Positive attitudes, pleasant thoughts, distraction, pleasing sights, topical lotions, and, yes, even humor can help manage pain.

Pain should be viewed as a signal to take positive action. It does not victimize you. This feeling of empowerment can build a sense of control vital to successful pain management. One idea is to practice self-talk. Don't reinforce negative statements such as "It's too cold to walk," or "I do look tired today." Think instead, "I'll wear my new jacket," or "Lipstick and a brisk walk will add color to my face."

Remember: You have arthritis. It doesn't have you!

Wendy Rivalis, who has had degenerative disk disease for the past 12 years, recommends these pain distractions:

☆Add a dash of drama. Envision a dramatic situation that uses that pain as part of the script. Pretend you're an actor playing a character in pain—a wounded spy escaping your captors, or a sports hero taking your team to victory despite your injury.

✷Savor the past. Conjure up details of a favorite pain-free, pleasant moment from your past. Relive the good feelings of that time.

☆Challenge yourself. Lose yourself in a game or project that requires your complete concentration. Try sewing, video games, or solitaire.

★Smarten up. Read a book or use instructional videos or audio tapes to learn something new. Learn to paint, speak a foreign language, grow herbs, or delve into spiritual practices such as of the Native American tradition.

✳Say goodbye. Imagine pain leaving your body. Be creative and visualize the details. For example, picture mailing your pain away. See yourself scooping the pain out of your body, placing it in a shipping carton, addressing the box to a faraway place, and sending it off.

✪Get competitive. Find a partner and play a word game, board game, or card game. If alone, do a crossword puzzle.

✵Call on your friends. Visit or phone friends. Focus on someone else's life instead of on your sore joints.

Pain Management

Let's Get Physical

Exercise, unlike medication, does not have to be taken with milk, does not cause allergic reactions, and will not deplete your wallet.

———

It can be performed according to your schedule and not only helps keep you moving, it makes you feel better in the process. It does, however, have side effects—reduced blood pressure, increased stamina, lowered cholesterol, lessened obesity, and natural pain relief. WOW! It also maximizes independence, increases flexibility…and reduces fatigue.

———

So, what are you waiting for? Get moving! The best time to get started on a program is now. It's never too late. Even if you're 90, it's still important to build muscle strength.

Even if you're 90, it's still important to build muscle strength.

Exercise

Tips

Before you begin an exercise program seek the advice and guidance of your doctor or physical therapist. They can help develop a specific routine that best suits your needs.

For Best Results—

✓ Balance rest with exercise.

✓ Correctly perform the exercises.

✓ Exercise slowly.

✓ Stretch daily.

✓ Know your limitations.

✓ Exercise when well.

✗ Do not exercise vigorously soon after eating.

✓ Wear proper clothing and shoes.

✗ Do not overexert.

✓ Use common sense. There is no gain with extreme pain when you have arthritis.

Pain Management

There are three basic types of exercise: range of motion, strengthening, and endurance. Each group has its own benefits and restrictions.

————

Range of Motion

Range-of-motion exercises are the foundation of any exercise program. They aim to move each of your joints as far as possible in all directions. The purpose is to increase or maintain flexibility and motion in muscles, tendons, ligaments, and joints. Flexibility is necessary for comfortable movement during exercise and daily activities, and to reduce the risk of sprains and strains. Flexibility is also important for good posture and strength.

Range-of-motion exercises are done gently and smoothly, three to ten times each, usually every day. Never bounce or jerk. To loosen tight muscles and limber stiff joints, stretch just until you feel tension and then hold for a count of 15. Arrange your exercises so you don't have to get up and down a lot. Always do the same exercises for your left side as for your right. Breathe naturally. Do not hold your breath. Count out loud to make sure you're breathing easily.

The

Exercise

Smorgasbord

> *Range-of-motion exercises are done gently and smoothly.*

Hand

1. Close hand into a fist, thumb on top of middle fingers. Open hand with fingers as straight as possible.

2. Place palm flat on table. Raise and lower fingers one by one.

3. Make an "O" by touching thumb to finger tips one at a time.

4. Crumple a sheet of paper into a small ball by placing the hand flat on the sheet of paper and gathering fingers into palm.

5. Rest hand on table, spread fingers wide, then bring them together.

6. Flip or flick ball of paper across the table, alternating the use of all four fingers with the thumb.

7. Curl fingers with wrist flat on table. Place thumb in palm behind index finger. Flip thumb outward as in shooting marbles.

8. Flip a light-weight magazine or folded newspaper off fingers by lifting fingers as a unit into the air.

9. Place wrist and fingers flat on table. Hold thumb with other hand to keep it from moving. Move each finger individually toward the thumb.

Pain Management

Wrist

1. Shake each wrist.

2. Palms together, arms stretched in front of the chest, draw hands in so that the fingers point towards the chest, moving the elbows outward. Keep the palms together at all times during this exercise.

3. Place a folded newspaper or light magazine across back of the hand and flip it from the hand.

4. Place hands and forearms on table, palms down. Raise hands up off table, allowing fingers to relax and keeping forearms on table.

5. Place hands and forearms on table, palms up. Raise hands, keeping forearms on table.

6. With arms on table and fingers loosely curled, slide hands from side to side. Keep forearms still.

Some more range-of-motion exercises...

Continuing the range-of-motion exercises...

Elbow

1. Sitting, bend elbows until fingers touch shoulders, then straighten elbows.

2. With upper arms at your sides and elbows bent, turn palms up, then turn palms down.

Shoulder

1. Sitting, shrug shoulders in upward, downward, and circular motions.

2. Standing, swing arms forward and upward, downward and backward.

3. Standing, raise arms to shoulder level and out to the side with palms up, rotate arms in a small circular motion forward, then backward.

4. Standing, keeping the elbows bent, place hands alternately behind neck and then the lower back.

5. Standing in front of a wall, creep up the wall with the fingers reaching higher each day.

Pain Management

Neck

1. Sitting, tilt head forward until chin touches chest, then tilt head back as far as it will comfortably go.

2. Sitting, remaining facing forward, gently tilt left ear toward left shoulder, then right ear toward right shoulder.

3. Sitting, turn face to left, then to right as far as possible without stress.

Hip

1. Lying on back, bend knee to chest, then straighten leg. Then, bend other knee to chest and straighten.

2. Lying on back with heels several inches apart and knees straight, roll legs inward and then outward.

3. Lying on back, move one leg out to the side keeping knee straight, then return to the starting position. Repeat with other leg.

4. Sitting with legs straight, bend body forward and touch toes with finger tips. Keep knees straight.

Knee

1. Bend knee as much as possible, then straighten. Repeat with other knee.

Those important range-of-motion exercises..

Let's finish the range-of-motion exercises.

Ankle

1. Sitting, bend feet up and down. Then, bend feet from side to side. Do not move legs.

2. Stand facing a wall about two feet away, and support yourself with your hands on the wall. Lean forward toward the wall keeping heels on the floor and knees straight.

Toes

1. Curl toes under, then straighten them out.

2. Place a towel on the floor. Gather the towel up under the foot using the toes. Do not pick up your heel. Repeat using other foot.

Remember: Gently. Smoothly. Three to ten times each. Every day. Never bounce or jerk. Stretch just until you feel tension and then hold for a count of 15. Don't get up and down a lot. Always do the same exercises for the left side as for the right. Breathe naturally. Do not hold your breath.

Pain Management

Start strengthening exercises if you already regularly exercise or if you can do the flexibility exercises for at least 15 minutes. Strengthening exercises ask your muscles to work a little harder than normal. This extra work demands that your muscles adapt. As a result, the muscles gradually get stronger. Strong muscles are important because they help absorb shock, support joints, and protect you from injuries. They improve endurance and allow you to safely walk, climb stairs, lift, and reach.

———

There are two types of strengthening exercises: isometric and isotonic. **Isometric** exercises are those you do when your joints hurt. Isometric means that the joints do not move. They are done by tightening up the muscle as much as you can by pushing against something that does not move. **Isotonic** exercises are those you do when your joints do not hurt. Isotonic means that there is movement in the joints. With isotonic exercises, you may use weights.

———

Start by doing no more than five repetitions. Gradually increase to no more than ten repetitions two or three times a week. Your muscles need time off to repair and rest.

———

Exercise—Grasp a tennis ball in your left hand and gently squeeze it five times. Repeat with your right hand.

A look at strengthening exercises.

> *Endurance Exercises: Take the talk test.*

Aerobic exercise, also known as endurance or cardiovascular exercise, is any physical activity that uses the large muscles of your body in rhythmic, continuous motions. The most effective exercises use your whole body and include walking, dancing, swimming, bicycling, mowing the lawn, and even raking the leaves. Their purpose is to improve the ability of the heart, lungs, blood vessels, and muscles to work as efficiently and effectively as possible. Weight control, improved sleep, strengthened bones, reduced depression and anxiety, and increased endurance are often the results.

If you have not been regularly active, start your aerobic exercise with no more than five minutes at a time. You can do this several times a day and gradually increase the duration of the aerobic exercise by alternating periods of brisk exercise with easy exercise.

The goal is to exert yourself moderately—not too lightly nor too intensely. If you do not want to calculate your pulse rate to tell how vigorously you are exercising, take the talk test. Talk to someone else or yourself, sing, or recite poetry, and see if you can do so comfortably. If you can't, slow down. Moderate exercise allows you to speak comfortably.

Pain Management

The many different types of aerobic exercise allow for variety. By alternating which exercises and activities you do, perhaps you can ward off monotony and maintain consistency—a common problem with exercise. Walking, swimming, aquacizing, bicycling, and low-impact aerobic dance are all good choices for endurance activities. Creatures of habit can find what works for them and then stick to it. Others can vary their routines.

———

Stair-climbing exercises are often discouraged for people with OA of the knee.

———

Before beginning an aerobic exercise, always warm up your muscles and joints with flexibility exercises for ten to 15 minutes. When ending the routine, always cool down for five to ten minutes with reduced activity and/or flexibility exercises. Do not just stop abruptly.

> *Walking, swimming, aquacizing, bicycling, and low-impact aerobic dance are all good choices for endurance activities.*

Endurance

Exercises

Walking

Walking is one of the most popular fitness exercises for people with arthritis. It does not require special equipment other than comfortable shoes, and it can be done inside or outside. In fact, walking in a shopping mall—mall walking—has almost become a sport in itself.

When Walking, Remember to—

✓ Warm up.

✓ Choose flat, level ground.

✓ Move your arms to raise your heart rate.

✓ Wear properly fitting shoes with shock-absorbing soles. Insertible insoles are available at shoe and sporting-goods stores.

✓ Maintain good posture. Keep chin tucked and shoulders relaxed to help reduce neck and upper-back discomfort.

If you have pain around your shins, do more ankle stretching and strengthening exercises before beginning. If you develop sore knees, slow your speed and do more arm work to keep your heart rate up. Fast walking puts more stress on the knee joint. Do knee-strengthening exercises.

Pain Management

Aquacizing

Aquacize is another way to use the swimming pool for aerobic exercise. Most facilities that have a pool offer some type of organized aquacize class. The Arthritis Foundation has an aquatic program designed specifically for arthritis sufferers. It is not necessary to know how to swim in this program. The foundation offers the opportunity to do gentle activities in warm water (Eighty-three to 88 degrees is the recommended temperature.) with guidance from a trained instructor. It also offers advanced levels for those ready for a more vigorous program. The Arthritis Foundation Aquatic Program (AFAP) usually has 15 to 20 people per class and conducts classes two to three times per week for 45 to 60 minutes. For information, call (800) 283-7800.

Aquacizing Tips

Protect your feet.

Keep warm.

Wear a flotation device for added buoyancy.

Endurance

Exercises

Endurance

Exercises

Research Results

Research indicates that exercising in warm water can reduce joint tenderness in people with arthritis better than simply sitting in warm water, exercising on land, or using progressive-relaxation techniques.

Swimming

Swimming is perhaps the ideal activity for arthritis sufferers. The buoyancy of the water lets you move your joints through their full range of motion and strengthen your muscles with almost zero stress on your joints.

To make it an aerobic exercise, you will need to aim for 20 minutes of continuous swimming.

Pain Management

Bicycling

Endurance Exercises

Bicycling can get you outside in the fresh air and sunshine—but it also subjects you to the traffic, uneven terrain, and concrete. Bicycle indoors on a stationary bike if these considerations seem too hazardous for you.

Outdoor Biking

When bicycling outdoors, be sure you have the right bicycle.

Your bike can cause more damage than good if it is the wrong height. Check the seat height by having someone hold the bike while you sit on the seat. With your heel on the pedal, straighten your leg to the bottom of the pedal stroke. If your knee is still bent, the seat is too low. People whose knees bend backward should leave just a little bend. The seat should be lowered if you can't keep your heel on the pedal at its lowest point.

Endurance

Exercises

Stationary Bicycling

For stationary cycling, proper height is also important. Follow the above guidelines.

———

Also, check to see that the bicycle is steady, the seat is comfortable and easily adjusted, the pedals are large, the frame allows ample clearance for the knees and ankles, and the handlebars facilitate good posture and arm position.

———

One of the most common complaints of stationary cycling is that it's boring. Make it interesting by watching television, reading, or listening to music or tapes. Many books are now available on tape. Instead of finishing a set number of miles, listen to so many chapters. Or learn another language via audio or videotapes. Take a trip to a foreign country by virtue of your VCR. Be creative and stimulate your mind as well as your body.

Pain Management

Low-Impact Aerobics

Low-impact aerobics means that one foot is always on the floor and there is no jumping. It does not, however, mean that it is low-intensity. Nor does it mean that all of your joints are protected.

You may have to modify the exercises according to your weaknesses in order for low-impact aerobic routines to work for you.

———

Perhaps the most important element of low-impact aerobics is the right instructor.

Choose an instructor who encourages everyone to exercise at his or her own pace.

Endurance Exercises

Crosstraining

One of the latest buzzwords in the exercise arena is crosstraining. To serious athletes, the term means excelling in various sports. To the rest of us, crosstraining means putting some variety into our fitness routines. A crosstraining program includes activities or specific exercises that increase aerobic fitness, muscular strength, and flexibility.

───────

Piece together a personalized crosstraining program by choosing at least one activity from each following category. Create a weekly schedule of which exercises you'll do on which days. Doing the activity more often for short periods of time may be the best plan. For example, if lifting weights, lifting a 10-pound weight for five minutes three times a day may be better than a 10-pound weight once a day for 15 minutes. Here are suggested activities:

Aerobics: Walking, fast walking, water walking, swimming, non-impact aerobic dancing, stationary and outdoor biking, walking on the treadmill, simulated or outdoor cross-country skiing , rowing, ice skating.

Strength: Lifting free weights, using weight machines, isometric exercises, pushing against elastic bands, resistance walking in water, using medicine balls.

Flexibility: Yoga, stretching, range-of-motion exercises, T'ai Ch'i.

Pain Management

Are athletes especially prone to arthritis?

Will the seemingly minor risks you take as you run, bike, hike, or otherwise engage in sports possibly end up sidelining you in later years?

Yes *and* No.

No—playing sports doesn't predispose you to arthritis.

Yes—certain athletic injuries can make it likelier that you'll get osteoarthritis later in life.

"*Sometimes it's exercise enough trying to live a normal, active life.*"

Homework

The idea that physical exertion, such as lawn work, gardening, and housekeeping, are exercise is new to some, but not to those who have been doing it for years.

It's true. You don't have to be a jock to get your exercise.

A 36-year old freelance writer from New York who has had two joint replacement operations says, "I try to swim laps two to three times a week, but I also do house, garden, and yard maintenance. Sometimes it's exercise enough trying to live a normal, active life."

Pain Management

Rest 'Em

When joints become painful, it's essential to rest them.

Rest does not necessarily mean putting them to bed, although it often does.

Braces and taping may stabilize the joint and provide support that allows the joint to rest.

Other ways include canes, neck collar, slings, and corsets.

Wedged insoles with a five- or 10-degree angle provide good symptom relief from mild to moderate osteoarthritis of the knee.

Whew!

After All That, I

Could Use a . . .

Heat Therapy

Heat is the most widely used pain therapy after medication. The idea that warm water is therapeutic has been around for centuries. An entire city was named for its hot-springs waters where people would come to bathe—Bath, England.

———

The two types of heat therapies are deep heat and external heat. The deep-heat therapy modality is ultrasound and requires a physical therapist. External-heat modalities often can be administered independently and include moist heat packs, paraffin, medcosonolator, hydrocollator, and whirlpool treatments. Your physical therapist can design a heating program specifically for you.

———

Heat works by simply increasing the blood flow to an area. It makes joints more comfortable and loosens them up. It also relieves pain and reduces muscle spasms sufficiently to allow each joint to go through full range-of-motion exercises.

Pain Management

M oist heat works best for most people.

I f you do not have a pad designed for moist heat, you can make your own. Cover a heating pad with plastic and then place a warm, wet (not dripping) cloth on top. Wrap this around the joint you are treating. If you have difficulty wringing out a towel so it's not sloppy wet, toss it into the washing machine on the spin cycle for a couple of minutes.

Sources —

AARP Pharmacy Service Home Care Specialog, One Prince
      St., Alexandria, VA 22314.

Medi-Mart Centers, 525 Third St., Beaver, PA 15009.
      (412)728-3851.

Ssssteam

Heat . . .

A House of Wax?

Paraffin treatment is used primarily on the hands—occasionally on the feet. It is beneficial for patients who have extremely tight skin or very dry skin. This treatment also puts heat between the toes and fingers which a heating pad cannot do.

———

Do not use paraffin treatments if you have broken skin—cuts, sores, or blisters—in the area you are going to treat. If you have extremely sensitive skin, you may not be able to do these treatments.

———

Small paraffin units can be purchased through a local medical supply store or ordered. They cost on average $150 to $200.

Sources—

Health Supplies of America, P.O. Box 288, Farmville, NC 27828. (800)334-1187

Hammacher Schlemmer, 9180 Lesaint Dr., West Chester, OH 45069. (800)543-3366

Pain Management

Do-it-yourself Paraffin Unit

You will need—
- ☐ 1 lb. of wax   ☐ mineral oil
- ☐ a covered container only for this use
- ☐ a candy thermometer   ☐ plastic wrap
- ☐ 1 bath towel   ☐ three 6"-8" strips of masking tape

Because you're treating yourself, you will only be able to wrap one hand at a time. Have all supplies ready and within reach. Fold and place towel on the table. Line towel with plastic wrap. In the container, heat the wax and four ounces of mineral oil over low heat. After 15 minutes, check the temperature of the wax. The thermometer should register between 121 and 130 degrees. Test the wax for comfort. If the wax is too hot or too thick, add more mineral oil. The first dip should leave a very thin film of wax on your hand. Then, keeping your fingers spread, dip your hand in the wax seven or eight times. Place your hand in the center of the plastic wrap-lined towel and fold the towel around your hand. Secure the towel in place with the strips of masking tape. Leave the wrap in place until the paraffin cools. Then, peel off the paraffin. To reuse the paraffin, pour alcohol over the used paraffin, blot it with a paper towel and put the paraffin right back into the container. Be sure to turn off the heat source when you're finished.

> *Maybe* that's *what Vincent Price was doing . . .*

Ultra-deep

Heat . . .

Diathermy is deep-heat therapy.

It uses tissue-penetrating ultrasound waves to heat up small areas of the body.

Diathermy is the only heat treatment that can penetrate beyond the surface layers of the skin to a joint.

———

In an arthritis survey, 81 percent of the people who had tried ultrasound said it helped ease their pain and stiffness.

Physical therapists usually administer this treatment.

Pain Management

✓ Take particular care when a patient is impaired and either may not notice a burn or may be unable to get away from the heat source if it becomes too hot.

✓ Remove any topical creams before applying heat.

✗ Don't apply heat to an area for more than 20 to 30 minutes. It might cause burns, and it will not add to pain relief because your body adapts to the temperature.

✗ Don't use heat if you have poor circulation, poor sensation, or increased sensitivity to heat. You might inadvertently injure your skin.

✗ Don't apply heat to a swollen, inflamed joint.

✗ Don't place heat directly on the skin; wrap the hot pad in towels. When using heating pads or packs, check your skin every five minutes for signs of burning. Add extra towels or turn the electric heating pad down if there are indications of burning. Be aware that temperature varies according to which device you are using.

✗ Don't fall asleep while using a heating device.

✗ Don't make your bath or shower too hot as it may cause dizziness and fatigue.

✗ Don't use electrical device that aren't UL approved.

✓ Adjust temperatures to children's sensitive skin.

✓ Heat should be mild and make you comfortable. It should never burn.

> *Warning! Hotter is not always better.*

More Cozy Accessories

Foot baths provide moist heat. Some have massaging action; others vary the speed of water agitation. These can also be used for the hands. Units are heavy when filled with water. Take care so you do not slip on any splashed water.

Foot baths can be purchased at many discount and department stores as well as health supply retailers.

Heating pads are available that are designed especially for the hands such as battery-powered mittens and mitts that can be heated in the oven or the microwave.

Electric blankets, electric throws or **joint warmers** are other heating accessories.

Sources—

Spenco Medical Corporation, P.O. Box 2501, Waco, TX 76702. (800) 433-3334.

Hammacher Schlemmer, 9180 Lesaint Dr., West Chester, OH 45069. (800) 543-3366.

SelfCare, 104 Challenger Driver, Portland, TN 37148-1716. (800)345-3371.

Pain Management

Treatment with cold reduces blood flow to an area. For a hot, inflamed joint or for a joint or muscle that's been overworked, cold seems to be the better choice.

———

Cold treatments penetrate farther and last longer than most forms of heat. They also reduce inflammation. Some people find it useful to apply cold to a chronically-involved joint or tendon immediately after exercising.

———

Cold Cautions—

Don't apply cold to one area for more than ten to twenty minutes. Remove the pack when the area has numbed.

Don't use a cold pack if you have any sensitivity to cold, decreased circulation, decreased sensation, or any cardiovascular problems.

Check your skin during and after treatment.

> *Place a towel between the skin and the cold source.*

> *Cracking your knuckles doesn't cause or increase your chance of getting arthritis. It may lead to swelling, however, so break that habit!*

Cold Cash Savers

Ice massage is recommended for some arthritis sufferers.

✓ Fill a plastic bag with crushed ice.

✓ Raid the freezer. Use a popsicle, a bag of frozen vegetables, or something else.

✓ Make your own ice cone massage aid by filling a cone-shaped paper cup with water and freezing it. Peel away the paper and—voila!—an instant block of ice.

Running Hot and Cold

✓ Some packs can be either hot or cold.

✓ After using heat or cold therapy, it's normal for the skin to appear pink. The pink should be uniform.

✓ If an area appears dark red or splotched red and white, it may indicate early skin damage.

✓ Blisters mean the temperature was too intense.

✓ Check for swelling or discoloration.

✓ Dry the area carefully and allow the skin to return to its normal temperature before putting on another heat or cold application.

Pain Management

Properly done massage has many beneficial effects. It causes the muscles to relax and an increase in blood flow. Muscles, tendons, and scar tissue are stretched, improving motion. "The general overall effect on the body is one of sedation," says Paul Davidson, M.D.

———

Darlene Cohen, in *Arthritis: Stop Suffering, Start Moving*, recommends a professional massage every week or every other week. This may seem like too much self-indulgence, but the physical benefits are convincing. Drug therapy is also expensive and people don't view it as indulgent. A professional massage can increase all-over circulation in the body and loosen the joints. Few other treatments do all that and feel good at the same time.

———

Say "massage" when people ask what they can give you for your birthday. A certificate for a massage makes a great gift.

———

The great thing about massage is that you can do it yourself. That's right. A masseuse or physical therapist isn't necessary. Research shows that people who try to help themselves (This includes self-massage.) usually heal faster and more completely, perhaps because of a sense of empowerment.

Massage: The best place to find a helping hand is at the end of your own arm.

> *Golf balls are perfect for massage.*

Par for the Course

Golf balls are perfect for massage. They're easily stored in purses, coat pockets, in the night table beside your bed, the glove compartment of your car.

———

Hold a ball in the palm of your hand and roll it over the area to be massaged. Experiment with different movements and tempos—rapid circular movements compared with large, slow, back-and-forth movements.

———

Put a golf ball on the floor at your feet while you're sitting in a straight-back chair. Place the bottom of your bare foot on the golf ball, and slowly roll it to massage your foot. If you find a sore spot, hold it steady with lighter pressure without moving the ball for a minute and breathe deeply. Use two golf balls, one for each foot, for simultaneous massage if you're well coordinated.

———

Slowly roll the ball between your hands to stimulate all areas on the palm and the outside of the hand between the bones. Two golf balls can be placed in the palm and slowly rolled around as you move your hand. Be careful not to overstrain or bruise your hands.

Pain Management

Massage your own back with tennis balls. Place a couple of balls close together on the carpet. Sit on the floor with the balls behind you, your knees bent, and your feet flat. Slowly lean back on your elbow. Gradually situate the area that needs massaging on top of the balls. Hold as you breathe deeply.

———

For hand and wrist massage, place a tennis ball on a table. Cover the ball with your palm. Roll the ball slowly between your fingers to stretch them. Roll the ball under the inside of your wrist to massage the wrist joint making small circular motions. Work up your forearm. Switch to your other hand. Similarly massage the top of each hand.

———

Throw in the Towel?

Sit comfortably in a chair. Drape a medium-size towel over your neck with the ends hanging over your chest. Grasp the ends of the towel firmly, with your head relaxed forward. Apply firm pressure downward to stretch your neck for five to ten seconds. Take a long, deep breath as you bring your head upward. Exhale as you apply the pressure again for five to ten seconds. Continue the exercise for several more times to relieve tension in the shoulders and neck.

Massage your own back?

> *Twenty minutes, two to three times a day, should be spent on self-help acupressure massage.*

Acupressure and How It Works

In acupressure, force is applied to a set of specific therapeutic points. Applying pressure to these points may interrupt the transmission of pain impulses to the brain or the pressure may cause endorphins to be released.

———

Exactly how acupressure works is difficult to explain scientifically. That it does work seems to be evident in the survival of the technique for thousands of years. In *Arthritis Relief at Your Fingertips,* Michael Gach recommends that 20 minutes, two to three times a day, should be spent on self-help acupressure massage.

———

There are 12 acupressure points that relate specifically to arthritis. These points are discussed by Gach. Although each point will feel different, some degree of soreness will probably be present with pressure. If the soreness is extreme, he recommends gradually decreasing the pressure until a balance is achieved between pain and pleasure.

Pain Management

The acupressure points at the base of each nail can relieve pain in the fingers and toes. If pain exists extending down into your fingers, relief can be achieved by putting firm pressure on the nerves that are close to the base of the fingernail. These points need about two or three minutes of firm, prolonged pressure.

———

The middle finger is the strongest of the fingers. If weakness or pain prevents the use of your fingers to apply pressure, your knuckles or other tools such as a pencil eraser, a golf ball, or even an avocado pit may be used.

———

Clothespins can do the trick. First, wrap the area with a washcloth or small rag. Apply the clothespin to the base of the nail or other point.

———

For more information contact: The Acupressure Institute of America, Inc. 1533 Shattuck Ave., Dept. 4, Berkeley, CA 94709.

Hang Pain out to Dry

To bi *or not to* bi . . .

Acupuncture

For thousands of years, Chinese doctors have prescribed acupuncture for what they call "*bi* syndrome"—arthritis. Now some U.S. doctors are trying the Chinese approach for patients who fail to respond to standard therapy. The technique involves inserting thin needles into pressure points. It is similar to acupressure except the points aren't "pressured" but are "punctured." The results have been moderately successful for the treatment of arthritis.

———

Taping

Some patients have found relief from arthritis pain that prevents their exercising by winding adhesive tape around their knees. This taping pulls the kneecap toward the center of the body. Researchers in England reported that 14 patients treated by this method reported a 25 percent decrease in pain. Taping may relieve the pressure on the joint caused by a poorly-aligned kneecap. In OA patients, the thigh muscles often weaken and contribute to a floating kneecap. The kneecap floats over to the stronger side. The uneven pull can create more workout-discouraging pain at a time when what you really need is to shape up those slacking muscles.

Pain Management

Hand Exercise

Tickling the ivories may be good for your arthritic hands.

Playing the piano can be a good range-of-motion exercise. Mom would be proud that you're practicing. World-renowned concert pianist and psoriatic arthritis sufferer Byron Janis whole "handedly" agrees.

It has also been observed that people who love music and enjoy playing the piano lose themselves in the pleasurable activity and forget for a time about the arthritis.

———

Typing is another, more moderate use of range-of-motion exercises for your hands. Maybe it's an opportunity for you to write the great American novel!

Make

Mom

Proud

Personal Care:

Hygiene

Shopping

Sexuality

Employment

Insurance

If Looks Could Kill . . .

Looks can't kill you, but the way you look can definitely affect the way you feel.

If you are clean and well-groomed, you feel better about yourself.

Make an effort to bathe, dress, and look your best.

Grooming may not be so easy if you are disabled by arthritis. Once-simple activities may now be difficult.

This section includes ideas that may help make personal care a little easier.

Personal Care

✔ Equip showers and tubs with safety rails or grab bars.

✔ Use nonskid mats on the floor beside the tub and suctioned rubber matting in the bottom of the tub or shower.

✔ Sit on a commercially-available bathboard or in a waterproof chair (Plastic lawn chairs work fine.) as opposed to the bottom of the tub. If you like to recline in the tub, a bath pillow can offer neck support. It should not push the head forward.

✔ Place all items for bathing close at hand.

✔ Soap on a rope can be placed around the neck or wrist for easy access.

✔ Liquid soap in a pump container may be easier on the hands than bar soap.

✔ Use a long-handled bath brush, bath mitt (can be made by sewing two washcloths together), or loofah sponge.

Rub-a-Dub-Dub, Safety in the Tub

> *When bathing, always keep your fingers extended, never bent.*

✓ Never wring out a washcloth or squeeze a sponge with fisted hands. Simply press the cloth or sponge against the side of the tub or another hard surface.

✓ For washing the area between your toes, try covering a yardstick with cloth or use a radiator-cleaning sponge.

✓ Attach a long, shower spray hose to make rinsing easier.

✓ Pat yourself dry or slip on a roomy terry cloth robe or cover-all and dry the natural way.

✓ Use lotion-type moisturizers, never oils. Oil can make the bathing area slippery and unsafe.

✓ When bathing, keep your fingers in an extended position, never bent, and use the palm for pressure.

✓ Take advantage of the warmth and moisture to do range-of-motion exercises while bathing or arm exercises while showering.

Personal Care

Dental Care

Electric toothbrushes and hydrocare devices can make dental hygiene easier. Any tool that allows proper, thorough, cleaning is acceptable. Choosing an angled toothbrush may make manual brushing easier. If gripping the toothbrush is a problem, the handle can be built up with sponge rollers, washcloths, or other soft materials.

———

Disposable dental flossers can be purchased at your local drug store. A floss holder can compensate for lost dexterity.

———

A tube squeezer or toothpaste in a pump dispenser can make applying toothpaste to your toothbrush easier. And using the heel of your hand or a pair of pliers often works just as well.

Say cheese . . .

Can we talk . . . Toilet Strategies?

Personal hygiene can present unique challenges to the arthritis sufferer. As you move on and off the toilet, be sure to open your fingers and use the palms of your hands for pushing.

———

There are many types of raised toilet seats which can prove invaluable. Be sure to keep in mind the shape that you need when purchasing one. An elongated seat will not fit a round toilet bowl. Padded toilet seats are also a good option as are armrest units.

———

Personal, portable urinals can free you to travel anywhere without worrying about proper toilet facilities. Premoistened wipes may prove more efficient than regular toilet paper for perineal cleaning. When self-cleaning is not possible or incomplete, bidets or attachable perineal cleaners are hygienic alternatives.

———

Feminine hygiene products now come in a wide array of sizes and absorbencies. Most are available with self-stick adhesive.

Personal Care

Deodorant sticks are usually easier to manage than sprays, but adaptors can be attached to spray cans.

———

Managing a manual razor can be tricky for anyone, not just an arthritis sufferer. Using an electric razor is recommended if you have poor grasp. Shaving down the leg, not up it, can reduce hair-follicle infections.

———

Soak thick nails before trimming to make them soft. Consider purchasing a special grooming kit or having someone else assist you if this is too difficult. A pedicure is good therapy as well as providing the grooming your toenails need. It can also help you avoid ingrown toenails.

———

Battery-powered manicure sets may be a wise alternative. Remember that nails may break more easily due to your illness or medication. Try a conditioner to reduce the brittleness of your nails.

Hair

Care

Stiff joints can make simple hair brushing difficult. Always allow ample time so that you are not rushed. Consider long-handled brushes and combs if shoulder movement is difficult.

———

Brush-type curlers require no handling of pins or clips. This allows rolling hair with just one hand.

———

Use the lightest weight blow-dryer or a free-standing dryer if heated drying is necessary.

———

Hair loss can be aggravated by dry heat so consider moist heat if medications or lupus make this a problem. Consider using moist heat rollers.

———

Sleeping with rollers in your hair may aggravate hair loss.

———

Short hair is an attractive option, as it allows reduced washing and drying time.

Personal Care

Putting It On . . .

If arthritis makes dressing difficult, joining a nudist colony is not the only option. There are ways to make dressing easier, which don't have to cost a lot of money.

✓ Buttons, snaps and zippers can be transformed—magically. The magic is hook-and-loop tape.

✓ Hook large paper clips over buttons to ease their insertion through the button holes.

✓ Sew on cuff buttons with elasticized thread.

✓ Try using a bent coat-hanger, Chinese backscratcher, expanding reacher, or dressing stick to pull up pants, straighten shirts, or retrieve out-of-reach clothes.

✓ Place large rings such as old key rings or curtain hooks, tassels, or medallions onto zipper tabs.

✓ Slide skirts around to the side for easy access to back zippers.

✓ Attach long zipper pulls to back dress zippers. Reach them more easily by bending over.

✓ Wear elastic-waisted pants.

✓ Consider buying clothes that are one to two sizes too large to make dressing easier.

✓ When possible, buy lined garments. They eliminate the need for separate slips or camisoles. Also, the smoothness of the lining makes slipping them on easier.

You're never fully dressed without a smile...

> *Most existing clothing can be adapted with a little creativity.*

Bras can present unique challenges. A stretch bandeau, sports bra, or undershirt are easier alternatives. They don't have hooks. Or, fasten a regular bra in the front and then slide it around; or fasten it, step into it, and pull it up. Or try a front-fastening bra.

———

If a girdle is necessary, look for the one that has a zipper or other features so it can be put on with one hand.

———

Half stockings or knee-highs are preferable to pantyhose. A garter belt and hose are easier to put on than regular pantyhose, which require a great deal of finger strength and dexterity. Another option is thigh-high stockings with rubberized bands at the top.

———

Put on socks with a dressing aid you can make.

Here's how: Cut x-ray film or construction board into the shape (not the size) of a ten-gallon hat. Attach a piece of cord through a hole punched in each side of the hat-shape's brim. To use: First, slide the sock on the sock-aid form and then drop the sock aid to the floor. Slide your foot into the shell and pull the sock on gently with the cord. Remove the aid. Remember, socks made from a silk and wool blend keep feet warm and dry without bunching or sliding down.

Personal Care

Clip-on ties can eliminate the fumbling and pain of trying to tie the perfect Windsor knot. Bow ties can provide a different and welcome change of style.

———

Wheelchair users find pantsuits warmer than dresses. Hip-length capes, ponchos, or serapes are preferable to regular coats in wet weather because they can be draped over the back of the chair to keep rain from collecting in the seat of the wheelchair and also protect the hands of the person pushing.

———

Having arthritis does not mean you need to invest in a whole new wardrobe. Often, special clothes are only needed during flares. Most existing clothing can be adapted with a little creativity and suggestions from PRIDE, Promote Independence, 391 Long Hill Rd., Groton, CT 06340. (860) 445-1448.

Stretchy belts eliminate the frustration of belt buckles.

Things to remember when buying new clothes:

✔ Clothes should be easy to put on and take off.

✔ Reinforcements where strain occurs eliminate future mending.

✔ There should be room for braces, splints, etc.

✘ Constriction, pressure, or discomfort is a no-no.

✔ Materials that are washable and do not need ironing are the most convenient.

✔ Front openings are easier to reach than side or back openings.

✔ Large, flat buttons are easier on the fingers.

✔ Soil-repellent finishes or sprays reduce the hand-straining scrubbing of spot cleaning.

✔ Deep hems, cuffs, tucks, or pleats can be let out or let down.

✔ Life's too short to spend it struggling with fasteners.

Personal Care

Some of These Things You Can Buy—

1. Rolling cart

2. Reacher

3. Hook-and-loop tape

4. Good heating pad

5. Safe bathroom

6. Good doctors—Keep a list of doctors' names and numbers in your wallet.

7. List of current medications

8. Support group—Friends and family count.

9. Positive, can-do attitude

10. Sense of humor

Top Ten Must-Haves for Arthritis

Great Gifts for Your Favorite Person with Arthritis

Massage certificates

Housecleaning-help certificates

Yardwork certificates

Paraffin baths

Special tools like electric scissors or large-grip vegetable peelers, etc.

Whirlpool tub adaptor

Remote controls for tv, lights, appliances

Healthy backpack

Travel pillow

Personal Care

Mail Order

Mail ordering clothes can be a convenient alternative to the physical strain of shopping. Many local department stores send sale flyers through the mail and are more than happy to take orders over the phone. Out-of-town companies send catalogues.

Mail Ordering Reminders

✓ Never send cash.

✓ Research company's return policy.

✓ Get the customer representative's first and last name.

✓ Check with the Better Business Bureau if you are not familiar with the company to see what kind of reputation it has.

Become a label reader. Take a magnifying glass with you when you shop.

Mail ordering clothes can be a convenient alternative.

> *"A man can be short and dumpy and getting bald, but if he has fire, women will like him."*
>
> —Mae West

Sexuality

Arthritis can present obstacles which get in the way of a healthy and fulfilling sex life. It's especially important to remember sexuality encompasses much more than physical intercourse. It involves our basic needs for intimacy, affection, approval, and acceptance.

———

Who you are will not change with the physical alterations that arthritis may inflict. In order to minimize negative feelings related to your altered physicality, you must be accepting, communicate, take care of yourself, and discard stereotypes.

———

Acceptance of negative feelings is the first step toward working through them. The goal is to replace negative feelings with a realistic acceptance of how your body has changed. There are many self-help books that address this subject. A counselor or psychologist can also assist if you feel stuck.

Personal Care

Ways Arthritis Can Get in the Way—

Physical problems—fatigue, pain, stiffness, vaginal dryness.

Side effects from medications—fatigue, impotence, risk for infections, weight gain, or bloating.

Emotional reactions—negative self-image, depression, or other emotional problems.

Relationship problems—from stresses of your illness or fear of causing physical pain.

Ways to Break Down Walls—

Communicate—talk, listen, share.

Take care of yourself—make it one of your daily goals to look your best. You'll feel better and so will those around you. Don't buy into the stereotype that people with disabilities or chronic illness are not interested in sex. Think about trying something new. Be creative.

Lighten up—have a sense of humor. Sex isn't work. The goal is to enjoy yourself and have fun. Discuss what feels good and what hurts . . . with words. They're easier to understand than smiles or sighs. Take turns giving each other a massage.

Set a signal—Agree beforehand to a signal for severe pain.

Oft said:

Laughter is the best medicine.

> *Some people credit water beds for making sex less painful and therefore more enjoyable.*

It's Good for You, Too!

Some studies have indicated that sex can be more than fun. It may actually be therapeutic. It releases endorphins—the body's own painkillers.

————

Use Your Sense(s)

There are many ways to have a fulfilling sex life. Touch, hearing, vision, smell, movement, and fantasy are all components that can be beneficial. Experimentation can be fun and helpful. Do not wait for your health-care professionals to ask if your sex life is suffering from this disease. Remember that sex is a daily living activity if you have problems. There is nothing to be embarrassed about.

————

If you are experiencing difficulty in a particular area, chances are someone else has as well—and has found a solution to the problem. Don't reinvent the wheel! Talk to your physician or your physical therapist.

Personal Care

A Checklist for Romance—

♥ Plan for sex just as you would any other activity.

♥ Choose a time of day or night when you feel best. You may be too stiff in the morning or too tired at night. Pace yourself beforehand, to avoid fatigue.

♥ Create atmosphere with candles, scent, or music.

♥ Share a warm bath as foreplay. It relaxes your joints. After, gently rub on lotions for pleasure.

♥ Time medication so that its relief occurs during sex.

♥ Experiment with alternatives to intercourse that involve less energy and movement, such as oral sex or mutual masturbation.

♥ Use vaginal lubricants if necessary. Avoid petroleum jelly and instead choose lubrications that are water soluble.

♥ Different positions may be necessary. The so-called missionary position can be uncomfortable if the woman has arthritis in her hip or if the man has it in his knee, leg, or arm. Have the less arthritic partner provide most of the body action. Use furniture for support and balance when both partners are standing.

♥ A personal vibrator can help if the hands are too weak for stimulation.

♥ Love, laugh and have fun.

> *To love others, we must first learn to love ourselves.*

> **Women's Personal Care: Listen with your palms.**

The performance of a breast self-exam can be difficult for women with arthritis in their hands. Joyce Guillory, Ph.D., the director of the Cancer Prevention Awareness Program at Morehouse School of Medicine, found an adequate exam can be done even if you can't follow the Cancer Society's guidelines to the letter.

If you are unable to "listen" with your finger tips, she suggests using your palms. Be sure to make the same small circular motions as you would with your fingers. Make sure you methodically examine the whole chest area—from sternum to armpit, collarbone to bra line. Try it with both hands. If you can't raise the breast by lifting your arm above your head, lift it with the hand that's not doing the lump-looking. This may not be as precise but it enables women to continue to take their health in their own hands—literally. That's important. At age 60, your breast-cancer risk is more than nine times higher than at age 40. At 80, it's twice as high as at 60.

Arthritis can worsen during the menstrual period. This is normal and is related to hormonal changes.

Personal Care

Employment and Arthritis

Arthritis can affect your work situation in a variety of ways:

✍ The diagnosis can halt a rapid rise to the top of the corporate ladder.

✍ It can lock you into a secure job because of wages and benefits even though the job is unsatisfying or stressful.

✍ It can force you to restructure your workplace or workday or work schedule.

✍ Some people may even deal with discrimination as a result.

I owe, I owe, it's off to work I go...

> *"Some days you tame the tiger and some days the tiger has you for lunch."*
>
> —Tug McGraw

Vocational Options

If arthritis prevents you from doing your present job, there are ways to continue working. Vocational rehabilitation and working from home are such options. The Vocational Rehabilitation Service helps people with disabilities develop different job skills. One out of every two arthritis sufferers finds employment through this service.

Vocational Rehabilitation services include—

- career counseling

- transportation assistance

- devices, tools, equipment

- licenses

- job training

- placement

Personal Care

For those with an independent flair and self-discipline, starting their own business may be an option. The Small Business Administration Office can give you information about their Handicapped Assistance Loan Program.

———

If this disease renders you incapable of continuing to work, you may be eligible for Social Security disability benefits. Social Security Disability Insurance (SSDI) and Supplemental Security Income (SSI) both offer specific incentives to encourage people to return to work.

———

Other Resources—

Center for Computer Assistance to the Disabled; 1950 Stemmons Freeway, Suite 4041, Dallas, TX 75207-3109. (214) 746-4217.

Job Accommodation Network, P.O. Box 6080, Morgantown, WV 26506-6080. (800) 526-7234.

President's Committee on Employment of People with Disabilities, 1331 F St., NW, Washington, DC 20004. (202) 376-6200.

Social Security Disability Insurance and Supplemental Security Income both offer specific incentives to encourage people to return to work.

> Look for a
> position that
> matches your
> physical
> capabilities.

Landing the Big Fish . . .

If you currently have arthritis and are looking for new employment, your main goal should be to try to prevent problems. Look for a position that matches your physical capabilities. Think first of what you would like to do regardless of your disability or limitations, then decide what you can and can't do, and try to assimilate the two into a satisfying career.

Focus on jobs that you can handle physically. Get a detailed description of all tasks involved in a potential job. Find out which ones are essential and which may be only marginally important. If you might have problems with some duties, figure alternative ways you can accomplish the tasks.

After narrowing your occupational choices, begin interviewing. For many arthritis sufferers, the dilemma of whether to tell the employer up front about the condition becomes an issue. John Parry, the director of the American Bar Association's Commission on Mental and Physical Disability Law in Washington, DC says, "It's a matter of intuition and judgment. If the condition is going to be relevant and obvious very soon on the job, you're more likely to need to bring it up. If it doesn't pertain to day-to-day functions, there may not be any reason to discuss it."

Personal Care

Employers can't ask about a disability in an interview if they employ more than 14 people. Nor can the employer request medical tests or exams until after making the job offer. Such legislation went into effect in 1990 with the federal Americans with Disabilities Act (ADA). This law only applies to people whose disabilities are "substantially limiting," and then only when the employee is aware of the condition.

If you think you could have problems doing the job, discuss possible accommodations with your potential employer. Focus on what you *can* do and accentuate the *benefits* you can provide. Don't subject yourself to any medical questionnaires, testing, or other screening methods unless you're offered the job or unless all applicants must undergo the same procedures.

Once on the job and your condition worsens, hampering your ability to perform, discuss it with your supervisor. Go prepared to suggest flextime, ergonomic changes, or other feasible alternatives. You increase your chance of a positive outcome by making him or her aware that accommodations are surprisingly affordable. If you're unsure how to restructure your work environment, an occupational therapist can visit the site and make suggestions. Local Arthritis Foundation offices may have additional information.

Focus on what you can do and accentuate the benefits you can provide.

It's Sometimes Unfair . . .

Unless the employer is aware of your needs, you do not have legal protection from discrimination.

If discrimination becomes an issue, keep accurate records with names, locations, times, and other pertinent facts. If you go over someone's head, you may aggravate the situation. Start with your immediate supervisors and have solutions available. If you don't get anywhere, then go to the next in the chain of command. Consider enlisting the help of a neutral negotiator. If you still haven't received satisfaction, consider filing an ADA complaint through an attorney or the Equal Employment Opportunity Commission.

The ADA states that an employer may not discriminate against qualified applicants and employees on the basis of a disability, as long as the employer has 15 or more employees. (An employee is anyone working 20 or more hours per week.) The law applies to all aspects of employment, including hiring, job assignments, training, promotion, pay, benefits, and company-sponsored social events.

Personal Care

Are you considered truly disabled? According to the ADA a party has a disability if she or he 1) has a physical or mental impairment that substantially limits a major life activity, 2) has a record of such an impairment, or 3) is regarded as having such an impairment. Major life activities include performing manual tasks, walking, sitting, concentrating, and interacting with others regardless of whether these tasks are required as part of the workplace responsibilities.

Legally, an employer must make reasonable accommodations for their employees. Accommodations are changes in a job or workplace that enable the individual to—

✍ Apply for a job.

✍ Perform the essential functions of the job.

✍ Enjoy all the benefits and privileges of employment.

> *"People who take control of their lives and their condition have better outcomes. Rather than feeling like victims, they feel better, require less pain medication, hurt less and enjoy greater satisfaction."*
>
> —Dr. Dennis Boulware

Reasonable

Accommodations

Examples of an employer's "reasonable accommodations" include—

✎ Creating part-time or adjusted work schedules.

✎ Restructuring the job—for example, removing mail opening as part of your job description.

✎ Providing assistive equipment or devices.

✎ Providing an access ramp or making the workplace more accessible.

✎ Changing the height of a desk.

Employers are *not* bound by law to make changes that would cause themselves undue hardship, defined as excess difficulty or expense. If the cost of the accommodation is considered an undue hardship, the employer must give you the choice of providing it for yourself or of sharing the cost.

The employer is not required to offer you special insurance coverage or benefits, only the same as he or she offers to the other employees. For more information contact the EEOC Headquarters, Attn.: OCLA, 1801 I St., NW, Washington, DC 20507. Section 920 of the EEOC compliance manual outlines who qualifies as disabled under the ADA law.

File any discrimination complaint within 180 days of the time the incident happened. Keep thorough and organized records. If your complaint is upheld, you are entitled to a remedy that will place you in the position you would have been in if the discrimination had never occurred. You may be entitled to hiring, promotion, reinstatement, back pay, and even attorney's fees.

> *"Any idiot can face a crisis. It's day-to-day living that wears you out."*
>
> —Anton Chekhov

Family and Medical Leave Act

Rest and Relaxation . . .

The Family and Medical Leave Act (FMLA), August 1993, allows employees to take up to three months unpaid medical leave per year if they are unable to work because of a serious health condition. You can take FMLA leave all at once, intermittently, or by working part-time. For example, you could use the leave to receive "continuing treatment" such as physical therapy. It applies to companies that employ 50 or more workers within a 75-mile radius. To be eligible, the employee must have been employed 1,250 hours in the previous 12 months.

———

Reasons for FMLA leave—

✍ A newborn, adopted, or foster child.

✍ A spouse, child, or parent who has a serious health condition.

✍ Your own serious health condition.

Personal Care

Workplace Ergonomics

E rgonomically-correct computers—

✍ Move closer to the keyboard. There should be a three- to six-inch space between your lap and the keyboard tray and desk.

✍ Keep your feet flat on the floor with your knees at a 90- to 110-degree angle and your ankles at right angles. If your feet don't touch the ground, a small footstool or box can provide support.

✍ Your fingers should touch the middle row of your keyboard. Keep your wrists straight yet loose.

✍ Raise or lower your desk so that you can sit with your arms relaxed, forearms parallel to the floor.

✍ The top of your monitor should be level with or below the eyes. The distance between your eyes and the screen should be 18 to 30 inches. If necessary, raise your monitor by placing a book under it.

✍ Reduce glare on the screen; it's fatiguing.

Take frequent computer breaks—get a drink of water or stretch every hour.

Computer Shortcuts

Macros—a series of keystrokes that you can record and execute or replay by pressing a few keys. Macros are helpful for phrases and tasks that you repeat often, such as typing your company's name or closing a letter.

Styles—a way to automate the way a document looks by recording specific codes and text. It can be used again and again.

Word-prediction software—software that suggests or predicts possible word endings after you have entered a few characters and lets you select the correct one.

VOICE-ACTIVATED SOFTWARE—software that responds to verbal commands. This is often expensive, but very helpful for people with severe arm and/or hand limitations.

Personal Care

Your Desk

A rolling, swivel chair with adjustable height and a contoured back is the preferable choice for sitting. Having all supplies within convenient reach is imperative. That means no undue bending, climbing, or moving of other items. Slanted desks and turntable desks may solve reaching problems.

———

Lateral files are easier to manipulate than pull-out drawers, which require standing.

———

Rather than using a hand-held telephone receiver, an operator's headset can free up your hands and eliminate neck strain caused by holding the phone with your shoulder.

———

For handling, sorting, and counting papers, checks, etc., consider fingertip moistener. This gelatinous material causes greater friction between the tip of your finger and the paper. Save hand and finger strain by utilizing a microcassette tape recorder instead of writing. Also, consider using a battery-powered letter opener.

> *Felt-tip pens require less pressure than ball-point pens.*

> *Poor lighting can contribute to eyestrain, stress, and subsequent fatigue and pain.*

✓ Poor lighting can contribute to eyestrain, stress, and subsequent fatigue and pain. Invest in a good-quality, high-intensity lamp and situate your desk as close to natural light (a window, a door) as possible. Remember, too, that glare on a computer screen can also cause fatigue!

✓ Magnifying lamps reduce bending and neck strain.

✓ Protect your neck and back when typing and copying. Use a stand or copyboard to keep the materials upright when typing. According to research, reading materials are best set at a 45-degree angle to your eyes. You can use a book or binder two to three inches thick and propped behind the work if you do not have a work stand. This angle keeps your eyes from having to constantly readjust their angle of vision.

✓ Enlarge type on the computer monitor with a lens or screen enlarger, which can enlarge up to 20 times the regular letter size. With calculators, use a rubber-tipped pencil instead of your fingers to operate the buttons.

✓ Distribute the weight of your briefcase with a shoulder strap.

✓ Short rests relieve fatigue. Spread your lunch hour over three 20-minute breaks instead of all at once.

If you have arthritis, you may need to be especially concerned about insurance because you may have higher medical costs than does someone who has no medical problems.

You may have more frequent medical bills.

———

A pre-existing condition is an illness or injury for which you've received treatment, or should have sought treatment, before the insurance policy was issued. Insurance companies characterize an arthritis sufferer as a higher risk.

———

An insurance company may give you an exclusion rider, which can mean there will be no benefits for that pre-existing condition. Coverage for the condition is postponed or the company will limit the amount it will pay during each year.

> *"Much more is known about stars than about rheumatism."*
>
> —Henry Haskins

Now that we have Medicare, we can enjoy diseases that once we couldn't afford.

Blue Cross/Blue Shield: In some states, Blue Cross/Blue Shield gets tax-favored treatment for offering affordable health-care coverage to anyone regardless of health history, age, or gender. After a specified time, perhaps six months, even a pre-existing condition is covered.

———

Medicare is a federal program for certain disabled people and those 65 or older who are entitled to receive Social Security benefits. For more information, call (800) 772-1213 for your nearest Social Security Office.

———

Children's Medical Services Crippled Children's Services Program is offered by every state. It provides comprehensive coverage to children with disabling diseases. Payments are based on the parents' income.

———

Medicaid is a health-insurance program sponsored by the federal and state governments for people who are disabled, blind, 65 or over, who have financial needs.

———

High-risk pools: Some states support programs that provide health insurance to people who cannot get coverage anywhere else. To find out if your state has one, contact your state insurance commission.

Personal Care

When Choosing Health Insurance—

✓ Read the policy and ask questions. This is easier now because new laws require policies to be understandable.

✓ Review your policy every year to make sure it's still adequate.

✓ Ask these questions—

> Is there a waiting period?
>
> What is my coverage for pre-existing conditions?
>
> What are my limits of coverage?
>
> Does it cover medications, outpatient physical or occupational therapy, or self-help devices?
>
> Are doctors or health-care facilities limited?
>
> What is the limit on how many dollars will be paid?
>
> Am I covered for a private or semi-private room?
>
> What is the deductible?
>
> Is the policy guaranteed renewable regardless of the number of claims?
>
> Will local hospitals accept this coverage?

> *Never hide a pre-existing condition. It will not be paid. If it's listed on your application and it isn't specifically excluded, then it's covered.*

Dirt Happens

Arthritis or not, dirt happens.

The dust on your coffee table doesn't care that you have arthritis. Neither does the soap scum in your bathtub, nor do the leaves that fall in your yard. You or those you live with may care, however.

Tackling daily home and garden chores can not only set those environments in order, it can also be therapeutic. For those of you who, like myself, equate housework with shock treatment, this idea may seem farfetched at first, but read on. I think many of the suggestions will prove beneficial.

Home, Garden, and the World

Until disposable garments are in vogue, laundry will be a part of life. Unless, of course, you can convince your Maytag repairman to do it with all of his spare time. Reducing your volume is probably a more realistic goal.

It all comes out in the wash...

✓ Use what disposable items are available, such as paper towels, paper napkins, and plastic tablecloths.

✓ Wash clothes before they are very soiled to avoid needing to scrub.

✓ Soak very soiled clothes before washing.

✓ Use a net laundry bag in the washing machine for delicates to avoid hand washing, or use a plumber's plunger (with holes cut in the cup) to wash and rinse hand washables in the sink.

✓ Plan your laundry room so it's user friendly. Store detergents, fabric softeners, and laundry supplies within easy reach.

✓ Have the washer and dryer raised to avoid bending.

✓ Special large knobs can make controlling the washer and dryer switches easier. If your laundry room is on a different floor, make sure you have a comfortable chair and a good book nearby. Don't go back and forth. Use time between washing and drying to rest.

Airing dirty laundry...

✓ If lifting a heavy detergent container is difficult, you can have someone put some in a small container, or scoop it out. Don't stress your hands. Liquid detergent may be more manageable.

✓ Line the hamper with a small plastic grocery bag and simply remove the bag by the handles if transporting dirty laundry from the hamper to the washing machine is a problem. The handles make the bag easier to carry and the bag makes for small loads. Don't overload the bag. It will make it too heavy.

✓ Sit while you fold clothes.

✓ Roll clothes in a towel instead of wringing them.

✓ Never carry a basketful of heavy, wet clothes. Use a push cart if possible to transport the clothes.

✓ Have a rack set up on which to hang the clothes. Make sure it is the proper height to avoid bending and reaching. Use old-style wooden clothespins instead of pinch clothespins when hanging clothes. Store clothespins in a bag that slides or hangs on the drying line, or even better, keep them in your apron pocket. Take advantage of gravity by letting the clothes fall from the dryer, rack, or clothesline into the basket.

Home, Garden, and the World

Etched in Iron . . .

✓ Iron only the most important items. Do not iron sheets, towels, or pillowcases. Hang clothes immediately from the dryer to avoid wrinkling.

✓ Choose an adjustable-height ironing board if you must iron that lets you sit in a comfortable position.

✓ Use a step stool or even a phone book to raise one foot when standing and reduce stress on the lower back, hips, and knees. Your wrists should be lower than your elbows if you're standing to iron.

✓ Select a lightweight iron with a comfortable handle. Cord minders can keep the cord out of the way.

✓ Use steam to avoid sprinkling. Use quick starch when possible or "permanent" starch which lasts through several washings.

✓ Do not bear down on the iron. Use both hands. Take long, even strokes instead of zig-zagging.

✓ Place the basket of clothes to be ironed on a chair near the ironing board to avoid bending down.

✓ Steamers can eliminate the need for ironing entirely. They simply steam out the wrinkles. A steamer can be used on hanging clothes, eliminating the need to set up an ironing board.

> *Do not iron sheets, towels, or pillowcases.*

Is it really necessary to vacuum under the couch every day?

Cleaning

Don't sweat the small stuff. If this has not been your life's motto before, it needs to be now. Remember this as you clean. Plan, yes, and organize, yes, and be realistic. Ask yourself, is it really necessary to vacuum under the couch every day? If you answer yes, skip to the section on obsessive-compulsive disorder.

✓ Make housework a part of your daily exercise. Crank up the music and pretend you're dancing.

✓ Save wasted steps. Assemble all of your necessary tools and cleaners on a rolling cart. Concentrate on one room at a time.

✓ Work at a moderate pace.

✓ Take frequent rest periods.

✓ Maintain good posture and wear proper shoes.

✓ Whistle while you work. It sounds silly but it works.

✓ Think happy thoughts. They may not make you fly like Peter Pan, but they'll keep you relaxed.

✓ Wear a smock or apron. It will create mobile storage, protect your clothes, and reduce later laundry.

Home, Garden, and the World

✓ Keep fingers flat and extended when dusting. Let the arm motion do the work. Use both arms to distribute the work for dusting and similar chores. Consider a dusting mitt. For polishing and cleaning, chamois may be easiest to use.

✓ Get rid of clutter! Streamline your accessories. If it's not there, it won't have to be dusted.

✓ A daily, light picking up accomplishes more than a monthly heavy-duty cleaning.

✓ Use cleaning products which do not require rinsing or scrubbing.

✓ Dust walls with a long-handled mop or broom. Use long-handled dusters, dust pans, and assistive tools when possible. To make your own long-handled dust pan, turn the handle up on a dust pan and insert a stick into it. Dust above doors, along baseboards and other hard-to-reach areas with a child's play mop.

✓ Keep a wastebasket in each room.

✓ Use a cellulose or sponge-rubber mop instead of cotton or string because they rinse out more efficiently. Self-squeezing mops are even better.

✓ Empty vacuum cleaner bags or carpet sweepers onto a damp newspaper. It attracts the dust.

Make it a rule, even if you're not Japanese, to leave shoes outside by the door.

> *What is worth doing is worth the trouble of asking somebody else to do."*
>
> —Ambrose Bierce

✓ When sweeping and mopping, use splints if you have them. Use pails on wheels that you push with your foot. To make your own, construct a wooden base fitted with triangular corner pieces to stabilize the pail and insert four casters under the base.

✓ Never scrub on your hands and knees. Sit on a low stool next to the bathtub and use a long-handled sponge to clean it.

✓ If aerosol cans are difficult to spray, select cleaners in easy-to-open containers, or invest in an adaptor. It can be switched from one aerosol can to another and changes the operation from a button- to handle-activated motion that uses lighter pressure.

✓ Keep mats by the outside doors. They'll catch dirt before it's tracked in. A shoe brush can also help. Buy one at a hardware store or make one by attaching four scrub-brushes to a solid wood base: two brushes lie on the bottom, bristles up, and two on their sides attached with L-brackets. Leave shoes at the door.

✓ Upright vacuum cleaners require less energy to use than most tank or canister models. They also allow better posture and can be used while sitting in a chair.

Home, Garden, and the World

Many people start the day making their beds, and as a result, misusing their joints.

> **With each sunrise, we start anew.**

✓ Begin making your bed before you get up. Use your feet to smooth the covers at the bottom of the bed.

✓ Have the bed raised (bricks and blocks of wood work well) to avoid bending.

✓ Locate the bed away from the wall to aid accessibility.

✓ Use stretch-fitted sheets that go on easily or use only flat sheets that don't need stretching at all. Nylon tricot sheets are lightweight and can be put on with one hand. They stretch without tugging. They're also easier to move on when turning or getting into and out of bed. They aren't best for extended bed stays, as they can cause sheet burn more quickly than cotton sheets.

✓ Comforters require no tucking and the down-filled types are extremely warm. Remember cold joints are stiffer joints. Electric blankets and light, but warm, bedding can keep you toasty.

✓ Use wooden pizza paddles to tuck sheets and bedding.

✓ Some people, especially children, may choose to sleep in a sleeping bag on top of the bed. In the morning, just roll it up or fold it over and tuck it into a closet.

Standing the Heat . . .

The first step to making life easier in the kitchen is proper planning. A conveniently-planned kitchen does not have to be large or expensive. It does need to be tailored to your specific needs.

✓ Get rid of anything you no longer use.

✓ Invest in a rolling cart. Shelia Goodwin, physical therapist and Clinical Director of The Workplace, Birmingham, Alabama, believes a good utility cart is essential in the arthritis sufferer's kitchen because it makes joint protection easier. Heavy items can be rolled on the cart. When a casserole is removed from the oven, it can be placed on the cart and rolled to the table. The constituents of a meal can be assembled on the cart and rolled to the table in one trip, eliminating several trips from the kitchen. Dishes can be collected from the table in one trip. Buy a cart with adjustable shelves.

✓ Store frequently-used items near where they will be used to eliminate steps. Do not scatter cooking utensils around the kitchen. Hang a pegboard near the stove for your utensils. For baking, store dry ingredients, mixer, mixing bowls, and measuring tools together. Keep the can opener near the canned goods and measuring tools in or near staple foods.

Home, Garden, and the World

✓ Plan storage so that one item can be removed without lifting and sifting through others.

✓ Keep heavy items as close as possible to the middle range of your reach to avoid lifting.

✓ Vertical storage is easiest. It eliminates stacking. Use vertical racks to store dishes, pans, and other heavy items.

✓ You can use palms for getting dishes out of vertical racks for better finger-joint protection.

✓ Drawer dividers create vertical filing within drawers.

✓ In cupboards, sliding storage devices and pull-out organizers reduce bending.

✓ Lazy Susans bring items within easy view and reach.

✓ Cupboard doors make good storage areas: Install semicircular shelves that bring out the contents as the door is opened.

✓ Expandable shelves reduce the need to stack and pile. They also can double your storage.

> *"It should be the function of medicine to help people die young as late in life as possible."*
>
> —Ernst Wunder

> *If you can't stand the heat, order in.*

✓ Magnetic clips and bins can turn the stove, refrigerator, and dishwasher into easy-to-see storage areas.

✓ Work areas should have sufficient space to work freely and to slide things out of the way.

✓ The height of the workspace should allow you to work without raising your hands to elbow level. Usually 36 inches is an appropriate height for working with short-handled tools and 32 inches for long-handled tools.

✓ Sit while you work. If you must stand, open a cabinet door and prop up one foot on the bottom shelf of the cabinet to relieve back stress.

Home, Garden, and the World

Handling containers without stress is important for wrist and finger joint protection. The first step to opening is to stabilize the container. Next, use both hands.

An example of this is to place the container in a shallow drawer, lean against the drawer, and use both hands to open the lid or release the top. Less creative, but perhaps more efficient, is a mounted jar opener. Many arthritis sufferers believe the different kinds of jar openers available are some of the best technology ever.

———

Do not use your fingers when opening a ring-topped can. Instead, slip a butter knife or flathead screwdriver under the ring and pry it up using leverage. Lever from the other side to completely remove the tab. A wet cloth or sponge beneath the can prevents sliding. Some manicurists have free fingernail-saving (fingers, as well!) devices that are made especially for opening tab-top cans.

———

To open frozen foods or other bagged items, place the bag on its side and use a sharp serrated knife to open the end. Never rip a box open with your fingers. Remember your hands are not bionic!

> *God gives us the nuts, but He doesn't crack them for us.*

Opening milk cartons can be damaging to your thumbs. Use the heels of your hands to push back the flanges of the spout, then switch to a knife to pull the spout forward.

———

Buy milk and juice in the smallest, lightest containers possible.

———

When removing large containers from the refrigerator or from a cupboard, try bending your elbow and resting the carton or bottle on your forearm. Use your hands for steadying.

———

Rather than using small twist ties to re-close bags and bread, use wooden clothespins or bag clips.

———

Use pliers with built-up handles to open paper cartons.

Home, Garden, and the World

Space cooking over separate periods during the day. This will allow you rest so that you can enjoy mealtime. Cook double or triple portions at one time. This provides several meals with only one preparation and clean-up time.

———

Use lightweight items when possible. Avoid stoneware. Use plastic dishware instead. Don't use iron skillets. Try one of the several brands of lightweight cookware, special microwave cookware, or even aluminum.

———

Take the easy route when possible:

☞ Use frozen vegetables, ready mixes, pre-measured and pre-prepared ingredients.

☞ If you must measure, measure dry ingredients before wet ingredients.

☞ Try one-dish meals, such as casseroles.

☞ Baking is an easier method of cooking than frying and it's healthier.

☞ Serve food in the baking dish.

Now, you're cookin'...!

> **The worst thing about accidents in the kitchen is that you usually have to eat them.**

Keep vegetables in their skin when possible. It's easier, and boiled potatoes in their jackets have more flavor than peeled, boiled potatoes.

———

Place mixing bowls on wet washcloths for stabilization.

———

Place a bowl in the bottom of the sink when mixing or stirring to allow the sides of the sink to provide rest and support. A whisk is easier to use than a spoon for mixing because it offers less resistance. When you select an electric mixer, make sure you can manage the controls easily, and can insert and remove the beaters without difficulty.

———

A simple nail in a wooden cutting board can be used as a "vegetable vise." You can place a potato on the nail, freeing the hand that would normally hold it so that both hands can share the task of peeling. A cutting board with suction cups can help stabilize the object you are cutting so your hands are free to perform the task properly.

Home, Garden, and the World

Avoid lifting heavy pots. Place a frying basket inside the pot of water when you're boiling spaghetti. Just lift the basket out when it's done. The heavy, water-filled pot doesn't have to be lifted. Be careful about dripping boiling water on yourself. Let it drain over the pot.

———

Sprayers can be attached to the kitchen faucet so filling pots with water can be done on the counter. No more lifting full pots out of the sink.

———

Clean implements as you go. Scald dishes and let them drain dry. Soak pots in hot, soapy water to eliminate scouring. There are pans with stick-free surfaces that are easy to clean up.

———

To aid lifting dishes out of the sink, make a ramp or "escalator." Hinge two lengths of eight- to ten-inch-wide boards together in the middle and finish with waterproof varnish.

———

The most functional type of faucet is one with either a single lever or levers on the individual handles, not the one with knobs you turn.

> *No more lifting full pots out of the sink.*

When washing dishes by hand, if you are right handed, arrange the dishwashing procedure so that work proceeds from left to right. Start with the dirty dishes on the left, then the wash water, then the rinse water, and finally, the dish drainer on the right. Air dry all dishes after rinsing them with hot water. The level of your dishpan can be raised by putting something beneath it.

———

Think disposable. Use foil pans when cooking if possible or line the broiling pan, casserole dish, or cookie sheet with aluminum foil. Also, use paper cups for muffin tins and plastic and paper products to reduce dishwashing.

———

✓ Replace hard-to-open drawers with magnetic catches.

✓ Add loops to drawers so they can be opened with the forearm.

✗ Do not pour from the cooking pan; ladle instead with a long-handled utensil.

✓ Tongs release food faster than a fork.

✓ Use elbow-length gloves to protect your forearms. Oven mitts allow your palms to carry the weight, not the wrists.

✓ Buy pots and pans with two handles so you can use both hands when lifting.

A standard-sized ice cream scoop is a perfect measure for cupcakes, pancakes, and muffins. Simply scoop the batter into the cups or onto the griddle—no more lifting and pouring from a heavy batter bowl.

———

Let technology work for you. Microwaves save both time and energy. They are usually simple and easy to operate. Electric can openers also save time and joints. Let a food processor chop and dice for you.

———

Choose your major appliances with an eye to controls that turn easily. Think personalized! For example, built-in wall ovens can be set at any height. Cooktops can also be placed at different levels. Smooth-top surfaces reduce the cleaning dilemmas of hard-to-reach nooks and crannies. Self-cleaning ovens are a good start—until the self-cleaning kitchen is invented.

———

Choose a refrigerator for easily-operated doors and convenient storage heights. Some people feel that top freezers and divided door units are the most convenient for storage of frozen foods. Add loops to refrigerator door handles so you can slide your arm in and open it.

Let technology work for you.

> **Don't be "functionally fixed." Look beyond an item's stated use. Be creative!**

✓ Bent coat hangers can pull oven shelves out for checking on a meal.

✓ Placing a cutting board over an open drawer creates a new, lower work surface.

✓ Substitute a pizza wheel for a knife for easily cutting many things besides pizza!

✓ Barbecue tools can also be used to reach into the oven to turn meats or stir without removing the entire pan. Be sure the length is sufficient for adequate burn protection—31 inches is preferable.

✓ A filled tea kettle can stabilize pots on the stove for one-handed stirring. Simply turn the pot-handle until the tea kettle stops it from swiveling.

Sources—

Good Grips , OXO International, a division of General Housewares Corporation, 1536 Beech St., Terra Haute, IN 47804. (800) 545-4411.

Wilton Industries, 2240 W. 75th St., Woodridge, IL 60517. (419) 666-8700.

Farberware, 1500 Bassett Ave., Bronx, NY 10461. (718) 863-8000.

Home, Garden, and the World

The Handyman Can . . .

① For quick household repairs, consider a **GLUE GUN**. They even come cordless for ease of operation.

② Basic **PLIERS** can be used for holding screws or nails instead of straining the fingers.

③ A **VISE GRIP** can be used for clamping rather than pliers.

④ Some woodworkers set up their shop so that **POWER TOOLS** do not have to be held by hand at all; they are held by clamps.

⑤ When unscrewing nuts and bolts, attach a vise to the **SCREWDRIVER** handle and use the vise as a lever.

⑥ Soldering is easier with a holding **JIG**.

⑦ **MAGNETS** can be used to pick up small screws and nails rather than fingers.

⑧ **OPTICAL MEASURING DEVICES** are easier to use than standard measuring tapes. Sync, Unique Merchandise Mart, Building 42, Hanover, PA 17333.

⑨ If you have a deep, rural mailbox, a slide-out **TRAY** can eliminate stretching and reaching for the mail. Contact Solutions at (800) 342-9988 for a catalog.

Sixty-two percent of arthritis sufferers enjoyed gardening more than any other activity.

Gardening

In a survey conducted by the Arthritis Foundation, 62 percent of arthritis sufferers enjoyed gardening more than any other activity. "It's not only something they enjoy physically, psychologically it gives them a sense of control that they may not normally have due to their arthritis," says Teresa Brady, Ph.D., the national medical advisor for the Arthritis Foundation.

* Space plants far enough apart so that a hoe can be used instead of a trowel.
* Magnetic bars help organize tools for quick retrieval.
* Hand tools must be light.
* Be sure not to overdo it.

Rather than kneeling, sit on a low stool with wheels, or plant in a raised bed. Use cushions or pads for comfort. A garden scoot lets you sit down rather than kneel, squat, or stoop. It can also be used for washing and waxing cars.

Weed after a heavy rainfall or, water heavily before weeding—this makes the ground more forgiving.

Seed tapes are an easy way to plant vegetables and flowers. Herbs and oriental vegetables are easy to grow in containers.

———

Digging attachments may be used with rounded garden shovels or digging spades. The swivel handle lets you dig up and turn over soil with only a one-quarter turn of the extension. A tiller attachment clamps to a digging spade or fork and provides a curved fulcrum to ease the task of pulling the tool out of the soil.

———

Hand trucks, wagons, or other rolling devices move items around safely. They also bring in groceries, haul tools back and forth, and are a means of carrying wood for winter fires.

———

Cutting the lawn may be a chore you choose to have done for you. If not, and you mow it yourself, use a mower that drives itself and has controls that are easy to operate.

The swivel handle of a shovel attachment lets you dig up and turn over soil with only a one-quarter turn of the extension.

> *"If a tree is planted straight up, it will be difficult for it to grow in a striking shape."*
>
> —Shen Fu

Gardeners in one survey said they believed this activity helped them achieve many health benefits. Here are a few bonuses they listed—

❀ Losing weight

❀ Reducing stress

❀ Keeping fit

❀ Improving mental health

Sources—

Breaking New Ground, Dept. of Agricultural Engineering, Purdue University, 1146 ABE Bldg., West Lafayette, IN 47907. (800) 825-4264 (voice/TT). (A newsletter for farmers with physical disabilities.)

Tools and Techniques for Easier Gardening, National Gardening Association, 180 Flynn Ave., Burlington, VT 05401. (802) 863-1308.

Home, Garden, and the World

It's a Small World, but . . .

Having arthritis can make any type of traveling difficult, even just getting to the grocery store. Simple operations like opening car doors, fastening seat belts, and climbing a few steps can seem impossible.

More complicated actions, such as negotiating a wheelchair in public restrooms and dragging luggage through an airport the size of a small country, can seem downright impossible.

DON'T GIVE UP! Having enough "will" can take you a long way—even around the world. Maybe the wag who ran out of energy before money needs some of our travel tips! Read on.

> *You can tell you're getting older when you're on vacation and your energy runs out before your money does.*

"*Happiness is activity.*"

—Aristotle

Planning is the first step for successful travel.

Begin by obtaining a copy of *The Directory of Travel Agencies of the Disabled* by Helen Hecker. If unavailable at your library or bookstore contact Twin Peaks Press, P.O. Box 8097, Portland, OR 97207.

Your librarian or local travel agent will have suggestions for other recent resources. Information about special tours, transportation, and other information pertaining to the area you will visit is usually available and well worth the effort of finding. The Chamber of Commerce at your destination is always a ready source of information. Bookstores have many kinds of special travel books. The Worldwide Web, if you have access to the Internet, is chockfull of data about every subject imaginable, including travel.

Home, Garden, and the World

Accommodation Booking Notes—

Ask about:

✈ The distances to the restaurant, pool, gift shop, front desk, etc.

✈ The location and convenience of the telephone. Some have phones not only by the bed, but in the bathroom too.

✈ Elevators, escalators, and stairs.

✈ Hotel-provided transportation.

✈ Accessibility of heated pools and hot tubs.

✈ Safety rails in bath.

✈ Room service.

✈ Carpet pile.

✈ Ramps.

✈ Emergency exits for handicapped.

Air travel is wonderful. It allows you to pass motorists at a safe distance.

> *Travel is educational. It teaches you that enough luggage is too much.*

Must-Takes

Name and phone number of your doctor

Prescriptions

Insurance information

Heating pad

Travel pillow

Portable nightlight

Folding reacher

Folding clothing-removing stick

Portable door-knob opener

Long-handled shoehorn

Fanny pack

Rechargeable razor

Lightweight travel wheelchair

———

We can put a man on the moon and phones in cars. So why can't we make remote-control luggage? Until we do, invest in the easiest wheeled suitcase you can afford and let others roll and carry it as much as possible.

Home, Garden, and the World

Up, Up and Away

✈ Book a direct, non-stop flight if possible. You won't have to change planes.

✈ Consider flying during the week; it's less crowded.

———

Airlines have policies for helping people with disabilities. They are usually willing to help in any way possible, but they do appreciate advance notice. Request any special services, such as diet restrictions, when you make your reservations. Reserve your seat ahead of time to avoid standing in line. Allow ample time. Arrive at least one hour before the normal check-in time if you require special service.

———

In the airport, use what's available—motorized transportation to the gates, skycaps, moving sidewalks.

———

A pencil with a built-up handle can be useful to trigger the overhead light and call the flight attendant after you are seated on the plane.

———

Stiffness can be alleviated with simple range-of-motion exercises or by getting up and moving around.

It's a small world, once you've made the long trip to the airport.

I've Been Working on the . . .

Most trains are barrier-free (another word for handicap-friendly). Some lines offer special assistance and reduced fares for disabled passengers.

___

For information on rail travel write for— "Access Amtrak: A Guide to Amtrak Service for Elderly and Handicapped Travelers." Office of Customer Relations, Amtrak, P.O. Box 2709, Washington, DC 20013. (800) 872-7245. Ask for the Special Service Desk.

___

At most Amtrak stations there is about a four-step climb to board the train. If you find it difficult to walk through a moving train, you may have your meals served at your seat or be seated in the food service car. Medication can be stored in the Amtrak refrigerator, but if you will need the medication between the hours of midnight and 6:00 a.m., you will need to provide your own cooler. Amtrak will provide the ice.

___

Amtrak has special swivel seats with fold-down armrests and storage space for a wheelchair alongside. Some trains have special bedrooms for a wheelchair traveler and a traveling companion, and a specially-designed toilet facility. Standard wheelchairs are allowed on passenger cars, but full-powered or extra-large wheelchairs must be transported in the baggage car.

Home, Garden, and the World

Bus Travel

The Helping Hand Services for the Handicapped allows a handicapped traveler and a companion to travel for the price of one ticket. Trailways and Greyhound also offer special services. Remember that bus aisles are not wide enough for wheelchairs, but they will assist you in getting on and off the bus. Non-motorized wheelchairs, walkers, canes, and other aids can be stored in the baggage area at no extra cost and are not counted as part of your luggage allotment. The driver will remove these aids at rest stops if you ask.

Before choosing bus travel, consider the following:

🚌 Can you sit for long stretches comfortably?

🚌 Can you get on and off the bus easily?

🚌 Do the food and restroom facilities meet your needs?

🚌 How long will you be traveling?

Items to take: Snacks, small pillow or cervical collar for naps, books, and games.

Contact: Section S, Greyhound Lines, Greyhound Tower, Phoenix, AZ 85077. (800) 345-3109 (TT).

Do range-of-motion exercises to alleviate stiffness!

Bon Voyage . . .

Cruises have become extremely popular in recent years for many disabled travelers, and they have proven a relaxing choice for arthritis sufferers. Extra-wide passageways, doorways, and elevators are just a few of the accommodations for the disabled. Some ships even construct personalized ramps for their passengers.

- Remember to lock the brakes of the wheelchair when you're not moving. The rocking of the waves can cause the rolling of a wheelchair.

- Always choose a cabin near the elevator and reserve a table near the entrance of the dining room if you have trouble walking.

- Take motion sickness medication . . . just in case.

- Confirm special requests with the crew on board.

Contact Cruise Lines International Association for their free booklet, with information from over 40 different cruise lines before deciding which cruise line is best suited to your needs. Obtain a copy of the *Cruise Guide for the Wheelchair Traveler* from to CLIA, 7 Battery Place, Suite 631, New York, NY 10004. (212) 921-0066.

Home, Garden, and the World

Traveling across the country? To the grocery store? Cars offer more freedom than any other mode of transportation. You decide when to stop. You decide what to see.

———

Your local registry of motor vehicles can advise you regarding vehicle modifications, as can the booklet *Hand Controls and Assistive Devices for the Physically Disabled* by the Human Resource Center. Traffic departments issue special license plates and parking stickers which may be useful.

———

Insert keys into built-up key holders for ease of use. A special cushion can assist getting into and out of the car. The inner surfaces of the cushion are made of a satiny, slippery rayon that slides easily. Make one at home with two thin foam pads and satiny fabric.

———

Lower-back support is necessary for any traveler, arthritic or not, planning a lengthy trip. If fastening a seat belt is difficult, attach D-rings to the driver's shoulder harness so that it connects to the middle seat belt on the right side. Check with the local sheriff's department or police station for modification approval. Many cars now have automatic seat belts.

> *Drive toward others as you would have others drive toward you.*

Wide-angle mirrors aid those with limited visibility caused by reduced head rotation. They fit over the standard rear-view mirror and increase the field-of-vision width to six lanes.

___

When you rent a car, request the features which will make your driving as comfortable as possible. Consider power steering, brakes, window seats, adjustable steering wheels, automatic seat belts, cruise control, lightweight doors, keyless entry or easily-operated door handles, and manageable ignition switches.

___

Reserve the vehicle four to six weeks in advance and get the confirmation in writing. Some cities have specially equipped vans modified for disabled drivers. For information about modified vans call Drive Master at (800) 889-6610.

___

Car-travel Checklist

✓ Keep all medications in the car, not the trunk.

✓ Take adequate snacks and beverages.

✓ Carry a hand-held lighted magnifying glass for reading detailed maps.

✓ Include an emergency kit.

✓ Rent a portable phone for communication.

Home, Garden, and the World

Around the World . . .

✓ Get shot (immunized)—call your local health department for more information.

✗ Avoid areas with unsanitary drinking water.

✓ Prevent insect bites with clothing, nets and repellents.

✗ Do not swim in fresh water where snails are common as they may harbor infectious bacteria or parasites.

✓ Get a check-up immediately after you return.

✓ Obtain names of English-speaking doctors at your destination before you arrive. The International Association for Medical Assistance to Travelers can help. Call (716) 754-4883.

✓ Respiratory infections and diarrhea are the two most common travel illnesses. Consider asking your doctor to prescribe medications you can take with you to have available in the event you do become ill.

✓ If you do become ill, always contact your doctor at home for a second opinion if possible.

✓ Carry a written list of medications and a doctor's statement explaining the need for the medications to eliminate suspicion by customs officials.

Traveling to different countries can be as painless as possible with a little extra planning. Do your homework. And stay healthy.

Rest! Rest! Rest!

- Be realistic. Scaling Mt. Everest might be out, but a helicopter ride in the Alps may be as thrilling.

- Start out **rest**ed. Don't get overtired. Alternate activities with **rest**s.

- Allow ample time to settle in at your destination.

- Prevent stiffness—keep joints warm and do your range-of-motion exercises

- Don't be afraid to ask for assistance.

- Use lightweight luggage. Pack lightly.

- Carry dollar bills or small denominations in the native currency for tips.

- Take comfortable clothes. Remember layers are best.

- Wear supportive shoes.

- Be flexible and considerate. If family members or friends want to do more strenuous activities or sightseeing, insist they go. Use this time for **rest**.

One of the most frustrating things with arthritis is that a flare cannot be predicted. You may plan ahead for physical difficulties and then not have any at all. Be thankful if that happens. It is always better to err on the side of caution than to find yourself miserable and wishing you had anticipated differently.

Children and Pregnancy

Mother Goose Gets It, Too

Arthritis is not confined to senior citizens. It is not even confined to adults. In fact, two hundred thousand children in the U.S. have some form of this chronic disease. The most common form is juvenile rheumatoid arthritis (JRA).

———

JRA is often mild, but can produce serious complications. The signs and symptoms not only change from day to day, they can vary from morning to afternoon. This is particularly frustrating for children who tend to have full schedules.

———

Arthritis is not inherited in the same way you got the shape of your grandfather's nose. Some people may be genetically susceptible or may have a relative risk for acquiring it. But arthritis doesn't follow Gregor Mendel's exact law of if your parents have it, so will you. Consequently, it's unlikely for two children in the same family to have JRA.

<u>Children</u>:

JRA

Play

School

Pregnancy

> **Three main types of JRA**

The three main types of JRA are:

POLYARTICULAR—which affects five or more joints

PAUCIARTICULAR—which affects four or fewer joints

SYSTEMIC—which affects both the joints and the internal organs

———

The most common features of JRA are—

joint inflammation,

joint Contracture,

joint damage,

and **altered growth**

Children and Pregnancy

Additional symptoms of JRA may be—

joint Stiffness

decreased activity

muscle Weakness

Some children with polyarticular or systemic JRA may have serious joint problems or develop other long-term complications, such as decreased growth

---

The long-term effects of JRA are not necessarily worrisome. There are good chances that your child will get well and suffer **no serious permanent disability**. Sometimes the symptoms just go away. This magic is called remission. No one can predict how long it will last. It can range from months and years to forever. No one knows why or how this happens.

> This magic is called remission.

> A positive attitude provides a solid foundation.

Parents do need to be aware that children with pauciarticular arthritis have a higher risk of chronic eye inflammation.

———

The treatment for children with JRA is much like that for adults with arthritis. It will probably be a team effort and include medications, exercises, nutritional eating, and coping skills. Adults and children differ in their emotional and physical needs.

———

Children are strongly affected by the attitudes of their caregivers, especially the family members. A positive attitude that focuses on what a child can do instead of can't do provides a solid foundation on which the child can thrive. Even young children need to know what the disease is, what to expect with regard to difficulties and treatment, and what their responsibilities include.

Children and Pregnancy

Perhaps the worst thing that can be done to children with any disability is to alter expectations in a way that separates them from their siblings, classmates, or other group members. If family members have chores, then the child with arthritis should, too. Depending on the severity of the child's condition, he or she may not be able to rake the leaves or vacuum, but might be able to babysit or fold laundry. The student might not be able to write in a journal, but can tape record the same information.

———

Remember Helen Keller! It was because of boundaries and encouragement that she had such influence in the world, not pity and coddling!

———

Be firm but be sensitive. During flares, the child may need extra help or encouragement. This is understandable. And don't forget they are, after all, children.

> If family members have chores, then the child with arthritis should, too.

"The human spirit is stronger than anything that can happen to it."

—C. C. Scott

Keep 'Em Active

Often children will not complain of joint pain; they withdraw or avoid the activities that increase the pain. Lack of use will increase the dysfunction of the joint so parents should encourage the child to participate to the best of his or her ability, but at the same time protect the painful joints.

Protection for children is similar to that for adults—

★ Make sure the child moves around or at least shifts positions every 20 minutes.

★ Discourage activities that involve holding the joint in a bent position for long times or that stress the joint, such as jumping rope, pounding with a hammer, or racquetball.

★ Ensure the child wears his or her splints or braces. With children it is especially important that the fit be precise. Over-the-counter devices are often made to fit adults. Seek advice and fitting from a physical or occupational therapist.

Play

For young children, play is an essential part of the learning process. Design their environment to encourage physical exploration if painful movements, stiff joints, or fatigue interfere with their natural desire to explore and play.

———

Bath time is an excellent opportunity for play because the warm water often soothes stiff joints. Shaped sponges, stacking toys, water guns and even rubber duckies can increase grip strength. Finger painting with bubble soap stretches and strengthens muscles.

———

Place toys up high to encourage children to extend and use their full range of motion in their shoulders and hands. Alphabet magnets can be placed on the refrigerator to see how high the child can reach.

Play is an essential part of the learning process.

> **Life is what comes next.**

Substituting an inflatable beach ball makes volleyball playable. Nerf balls are also excellent substitutes for basketballs, footballs, and baseballs because of their light weight.

Riding toys, such as bikes, trikes, and big wheels encourage full knee extension and strengthen leg muscles if the seat is raised to an appropriate height.

Lying on scooter boards and on oversized balls enhances balance and strengthens neck muscles.

Positioning toys on slanted tables or on upright magnetic boards can encourage wrist extension.

Children and Pregnancy

Enlarged handles, such as joysticks, can aid grasp. Microsoft makes an oversized, brightly colored computer mouse.

———

Mandatory rest periods are another difference between adult and juvenile arthritis. They are not as necessary for children. Because children tend to rest when they're tired, they should be encouraged to be as active as possible when their joints don't hurt too badly so that they can build up endurance.

———

Activities that should be encouraged which build up endurance are swimming, bicycling, walking, low-impact aerobics, and jazzercise.

> "Mouse—
> an animal which strews its path with fainting women."
>
> —Ambrose Bierce

> Life is a series of relapses and recoveries.

Keep 'Em Interested

Susan Wright, an occupational therapist in the pediatric rheumatology department of the University of Kansas Medical Center, suggests—

- First, **warm** the child's muscles with a heat pack or heated towel.

- **Discourage** bouncing and speed in the exercise.

- During a flare, **skip** the day's workout or **decrease** the amount of resistance and number of repetitions until she or he feels better.

- Make exercise, like bicycling, a **family affair**.

- Make a chart of exercise goals and record **progress** with incentives for reaching goals. Include goals for each member of the family to take pressure off the child. If the child is frustrated by not being able to do certain activities or sports, **encourage** experimentation with new activities.

- Make sure exercises are done **correctly**. Mild discomfort shouldn't last longer than two hours. Severe pain means stop.

Children and Pregnancy

The least physically restrictive school environment is preferable for the arthritic student and is also mandated by Public Law 94-142. This law states that all schools must provide modifications for children with disabilities.

———

The needs for children with arthritis might include tape recorders, typewriters, physical and occupational therapy, and special transportation.

———

Open communication with school personnel is an invaluable tool. Because the child's abilities often fluctuate from day to day, and because the teacher is a key factor in the child's success, the teacher needs to be educated about arthritis.

———

A pamphlet, When Your Student Has Arthritis, is available from your local Arthritis Foundation. It's a must!

Get your child's school day off to a good start.

Coping at School

You can help get your child's school day off to a good start by setting the tempo at home in the morning. Take a little extra time with him or her. Help the child limber up joints and muscles by stretching or soaking them in warm water.

———

Plan so the morning is not rushed.

———

Keep two sets of books—one at home and one at school. This eliminates lugging heavy backpacks.

———

Ask physical education instructors to design activities appropriate for your child.

Children and Pregnancy

Many people do not hesitate to treat the physical symptoms with medications and physical therapy, but they balk at treating the non-physical side. Trained counselors can be recommended by your physician and may prove to be an essential link in the treatment chain.

———

Depending on the age of the child, the physical aspect of dealing with the disease may not be the most difficult to handle; the emotional aspect may be. The key to dealing healthily with emotions, according to Daphne Finlay of the Alabama Institute of Pastoral Counseling and certified play therapist, is to express them. "Parents should create safe outlets for the communication of 'negative' emotions as well as 'positive' emotions. Above all do not be afraid to seek assistance."

> The physical aspect may not be the most difficult to handle; the emotional aspect may be.

> **Teasers look for a reaction so don't reward them with one.**

If **teasing** is a problem, equip your child with the necessary ammunition. Practice and role play potential situations with your child. This helps remove fear. Teach that **appearing calm** is often the best offense. Don't look upset. That's what teasers want. Teasers look for a **reaction** so don't reward them with one. Face the teaser with hands on hips and keep **direct eye contact**. Appear calm while responding appropriately. Later, approach the teaser alone and discuss the incident. If teasing becomes severe, though, parents and teachers may need to get **involved**. Encourage the child to work it out him or herself first.

Schedule time alone with healthy siblings. Listen to them with an accepting attitude. Unexpressed feelings don't disappear. They can resurface in unhealthy ways. Signs of this may include such things as depression, hostility, or sickness. Arrange for them to be with peers with similar family situations.

Children and Pregnancy

F.Y.I. for your kid:

JRA is not **contagious**.

Rarely does more than **one child** in a family get arthritis.

More **girls** than boys get arthritis.

Sleeping in a warm, cozy **sleeping bag** can decrease morning stiffness.

Most kids respond better to **heat therapy** than cold therapy.

A mother should be like a quilt—keep the children warm but don't smother them.

> "The entire population of the universe, with one trifling exception, is composed of others."

A Bun in the Oven . . .

Ideally, the decision to become pregnant should be deliberate. As with any major life decision, it should be made when not under stress.

———

Questions to ask yourself include—

- Why do I want to get pregnant?

- Am I expecting the baby to fill a void in my life?

- Will I have help during my pregnancy if I need it?

- Am I financially, personally, and emotionally stable?

Children and Pregnancy

Pregnancy, especially with rheumatoid arthritis, may cause improvement. This is not a reason to become pregnant, however. Lupus may stay the same, improve, or flare. If your illness does improve during pregnancy, it may flare soon after the baby's birth.

————

Because the world is not ideal, pregnancy often happens unplanned. Having an abortion will not prevent a flare.

————

Normal physical changes may affect your joints and muscles in the following ways—

❣ Joints may become looser.

❣ Muscle spasms in the back may occur.

❣ Water weight may increase stiffness.

————

Consult a physician as soon as possible upon discovering your pregnancy and develop a treatment plan.

> During pregnancy, normal physical changes may affect your joints.

> Consult your doctor about the effect of your medication on the baby.

Decisions about Breast-Feeding...

Most medications taken for arthritis are passed to the baby through the mother's milk.

Ibuprofen seems to be a possible exception.

Consult your OB-GYN for more information about this and all medications you may consider taking during this time.

Eating for Wellness

Eating for Wellness

It's unanimous! Researchers recommend a good, well-balanced diet for arthritis sufferers.

Why? Because there is a link between diet and health. Scientists now know that diet may serve as a risk factor by increasing your chances for developing certain kinds of arthritis. Diet may also change the way your body's defenses—the immune system—react in certain kinds of arthritis that involve inflammation. Preliminary studies with animals and a small number of people suggest, but do not prove, that changes in the diet may help.

That's the good news. The bad news is that until the evidence is more solid, the only recommended dietary changes your doctor is likely to make are for weight control.

> "An endocrinologist once told me that the best procedure when business must be combined with eating is to watch your victim's ear lobes and feed him rare beef. When his lobes turn ruddy, make your proposition . . . and quickly!"
>
> —M.F.K. Fisher

"It is a sacred duty for all the fathers and mothers of the world to forbid coffee to their children with great severity, if they do not wish to produce dried-up little monsters."

—Brillat-Savarin

There are several connections between food and specific forms of arthritis. Gout, osteoporosis, and Reiter's syndrome are examples. A painful attack of gout can be triggered by foods with high levels of a chemical called purine. One of the effects of gout is an impaired ability to rid the body of or use up the purines. Therefore, foods with high levels of purine can aggravate the symptoms. Luckily, gout is a form of arthritis that can be effectively treated by medication. The medication almost eliminates the need to change your diet, but your doctor may suggest you increase your fluid intake because additional fluids assist the body in flushing out the purines.

———

Foods high in purine include wine, anchovies, beer, gravies, and liver. Other foods which may need to be avoided: mushrooms, asparagus, spinach, artichokes, peas, and beans. Bourbon may also need to be avoided; vodka may be a better substitute for an occasional indulgence.

———

Calcium, caffeine, and alcohol play a part in bone strength. Too little calcium or too much alcohol contributes to weak bones and increases your chances for getting osteoporosis. A lifetime of coffee drinking may also decrease bone density. With osteoporosis, bones are brittle, break easily, and repair slowly.

Eating for Wellness

A form of arthritis called Reiter's syndrome seems to develop after a person's exposure to food or water contaminated by certain bacteria. This rare type of arthritis indicates a defect in the immune system which increases the likelihood of developing arthritis.

———

Okay, so you know you should eat a balanced diet, but knowing it and doing it are two different things. Eat a variety of foods from the four basic food groups: grain products, vegetables and fruit, milk products, and meats and meat substitutes. If you do this, chances are you're getting most of the vitamins and minerals you need. Choose a supplement, if you want one, with 50 percent to 100 percent of the recommended daily allowance. There's no reason to take megadoses of vitamins unless ordered by your doctor.

———

In developed nations, too much alcohol and saturated fat are the most common nutritional excesses. Approximately 40 percent of total calories in the American diet come from fat. Carbohydrates, protein, and fat are converted into fat when they are ingested in excess of energy demands. One gram of fat can release nine calories as compared with four calories potentially released by either one gram of protein or one gram of carbohydrate.

Grain products, vegetables and fruit, milk products, and meats and meat substitutes...

> *A healthy weight is important to people with arthritis.*

Weight is a problem for some people—either gaining it or losing it. Maintaining a healthy weight is important to people with arthritis because it balances the stress on your joints and allows you to feel better which makes you a better manager of your health. To lose weight, you will need to become more active and alter your eating habits. To gain weight, you will also need to alter your eating patterns and attitude toward food.

To Lose Weight—

- Be patient. Set your goal to lose weight gradually, one or two pounds a month. Identify specific steps you will take to do this. Instead of saying to yourself, "I need to lose ten pounds now." say, "Gradually losing weight helps me keep it off for good."

- Eat less fat; learn to count fat grams.

- Eat slowly.

- Drink lots of water.

- Avoid skipping meals.

- Snack sensibly between meals.

- Eat frequent, small meals.

- Chew your food well. Food is enjoyable. This also decreases the burden on your digestive system.

- Relax for half an hour before you eat.

Eating for Wellness

To Gain Weight

- Eat smaller meals frequently during the day.

- Snack on high-calorie beverages such as shakes and malts. Eat high-protein foods.

- Use milk to prepare creamed dishes with meat, fish or poultry. Add milk or milk powder to sauces, gravies, cereals, soups, and casseroles.

- Add meat to salads, soups, and casseroles.

- Melt cheese on vegetables.

- Add butter or margarine to dishes.

- Don't skip meals.

- Use protein, vitamin, and mineral supplements if needed.

You Say it Tastes Like Sand . . .

If food doesn't taste good because of medications you may overcompensate with salt. Be careful because this can cause water retention or bloating which can increase blood pressure.

———

Enhance flavors by experimenting with lemon juice, herbs, spices and other seasonings.

———

Modify recipes to include a wide variety of ingredients to make food look and taste more appealing.

———

Chew your food well. This will allow the food to remain in your mouth longer and stimulate your taste buds more.

Eating for Wellness

Dining out can be both enjoyable and healthy. Remember these suggestions for healthier eating—

✓ Select restaurants that offer a variety of foods and flexible preparation. Ask what is in a dish and how it is prepared. Request healthier preparation methods.

✓ Plan ahead what type of food you will eat and how much. Order before hearing others order so that you aren't tempted to change yours.

✓ Select items low in fat, sodium, and sugar.

✓ Request dressings, sauces, and gravies on the side.

✓ Choose fish or poultry over red meat.

✓ Avoid breaded, fried, sauteed, or creamy dishes.

✓ Choose dishes whose ingredients are listed.

✓ Order à la carte instead of a whole dinner.

✓ For fast food, choose salads with dressing on the side, baked potatoes instead of fries, juice or water, not soda, and frozen yogurt instead of ice cream.

———

Consult the *Healthy Eater's Guide to Family and Chain Restaurants* and *The Restaurant Companion*, by Hope Warshaw, R.D.

Your table, Monsieur et Madame . . .

Make Mine Hot and Sour . . .

When eating Chinese food, eat more rice than entree. Select dishes with lighter-colored sauces if salt conscious. They have less soy sauce, oyster sauce, hoisin sauce, and black bean sauce, which are on the heavier, saltier side. Also, request that the food be prepared without MSG (monosodium glutamate). Eat with chopsticks—especially if you're not good at it! This will actually slow down your eating and may help your realize you're full before you overeat.

———

Healthier Selections—

Wonton soup, and hot and sour soup

Steamed dumplings

Entrees in light brown or lobster sauce

Chinese pancakes

Entrees with lots of vegetables

Vegetable or shrimp lo mein

Pineapple chunks or lychee nuts

Steamed white rice

———

Only occasionally indulge yourself with egg rolls and spring rolls, fried wontons, the pupu platter, sweet and sour entrees (meat is battered and fried), entrees with nuts or duck, crispy whole fish, fried fruit, and fried rice.

Eating for Wellness

In Mexican restaurants, stay away from the cheese and sour cream-laden dishes. Choose the lighter options such as fajitas, either chicken or vegetable. Ask for corn tortillas rather than flour. Get warmed tortillas and salsa instead of fried chips.

Healthier Selections—

Steamed corn tortillas with salsa

Black bean soup

Gazpacho

Bean burritos

Chicken or vegetable fajitas

Mexican rice

Pinto or black beans

Flan

Only occasionally choose chips with guacamole, nachos, chili con queso, quesadillas, chimichangas, other entrees made with fried tortillas, refried beans, sopapillas, chile rellenos, and enchiladas. Ask for them without melted cheese on the top. Use mole′ or salsa as a substitute.

Gimme a fajita. Hold the guacamole . . .

When in Rome, easy on the pepperoni . . .

When eating Italian, opt for the tomato-based sauces, not the cream sauces. Go light on the cheeses.

Healthier Selections—

Marinated mushrooms

Italian bread

Clams or mussels steamed in white wine

Antipasto (easy on the salami, pastrami and oil)

Minestrone soup

Wine

Pasta with marinara sauce

Bolognese, vegetable, or seafood sauces

Veal or chicken cacciatore

Pizza with vegetable toppings

Italian ice

Only occasionally choose garlic bread, Caesar salad, fried calamari, stuffed pastas (ravioli, cannelloni, tortellini), scampi-style entrees, parmigiana-style or saltimbocca-style entrees, canaille, and tortoni. Rarely order pizza with pepperoni, sausage, meatballs, or extra-cheese toppings or double crust. Skip the cheese and get extra marinara sauce.

Eating for Wellness

Just because a diet is "unproven" doesn't necessarily mean it doesn't work. It means the claims are still being studied or have not yet been proven effective or safe. With arthritis, what works for you may not work for someone else. Keep this in mind with the various diets. Even though a diet may not be proven to work for a large percentage of people, if it works for you, who cares what the numbers say! A word of caution—do not try diets that eliminate entire groups of foods or stress only a few foods. Remember healthy eating always includes balance.

When Considering a Special Diet—

✓   Research it.

✓   Determine what caused the results. Could something aside from the food have caused the results—positive thinking, reduced activity, coincidence?

✓   Was the study conducted scientifically? One person's improving does not scientific evidence make.

✓   Don't hesitate to consult with your physician or other health professional for advice.

✓   Weigh the slight chance that the diet will offer results against cost, inconvenience, and side effects.

Good luck! Maybe you'll stumble on something that works for you.

Just because you can't see it, doesn't mean . . .

> *Certain foods aggravate arthritis...*

NO ONE ADVISES CONTINUOUS FASTING AS TREATMENT!

A study presented in 1988 in *Annals of Rheumatic Diseases* concluded that certain foods do aggravate arthritis. The problem is that these "certain foods" change from one person to the next.

Diet studies that include a period of fasting show that arthritis almost always improves in the absence of food. This finding suggests there is some aggravating factor in food.

And food is necessary for life as a healthy diet is necessary for healthy living. Don't avoid eating because you think that it will improve arthritis. It could very well complicate the arthritis and create other problems for you.

Food Allergies and Arthritis

Food allergies seem to be at the root of some types of arthritis. Whether it is a true allergy or a food intolerance does not matter to the patient. The outcome is the same—pain.

Somehow a person's intestinal wall becomes permeable— perhaps because of inflammation, bacterial overgrowth, an allergic tendency, or even taking anti-inflammatory drugs. The permeations allow large molecules of a food, like milk, through the intestinal membrane and into the bloodstream. There the body's immune system treats the molecules of milk as though they were harmful invaders such as bacteria or viruses.

Terry Phillips, Ph.D., the director of the immunogenetics and immunochemistry laboratory at George Washington University, said, "In response to the milk molecules (called antigens), the body's immune cells develop antibodies which can latch onto the milk antigens. These are absorbed through the gut and become creatures called circulating immune complexes, which go around the body's bloodstream until they can find a good place to be deposited. Circulating immune complexes may stick to blood-vessel walls, where they cause hives and vasculitis. Or a very common place for them to go is into the joints, especially if the joint is already damaged by an arthritic flare-up."

More Food Allergies and Arthritis

In the joint, the immune complexes lie on the synovium, the tissue lining the joint capsule. There they attract what Dr. Phillips called the "garbage-collection cells"—macrophages—which gobble up the immune complexes and tear up the joint tissue as well, causing localized inflammation.

It's also possible for a food antigen to travel alone to a joint, and there be attacked by antibodies that are on the surface of mast cells in the synovium. When this happens, the mast cells detonate like microscopic bombs, releasing a spray of inflammatory biochemicals into your joint that destroys the milk antigen and perhaps damages a few joint cells in the process.

A similar allergic response can occur in almost any organ in the body," said Dean Metcalfe, M.D., head of the mast-cell physiology section of the National Institute of Allergy and Infectious Disease in Bethesda, Maryland. "A person's genetic predisposition may determine which organs are targeted for an allergic response."

Eating for Wellness

Allergies and Rheumatoid Arthritis

Doctors disagree about how RA sufferers have conditions aggravated by food. Some of them believe the figure is as low as five percent or less. Other physicians argue that it may be as much as 30 percent.

———

Do RA sufferers have more allergies in general? Research seems to indicate that they do not. Allergic disease is no more common in people with RA than it is in the general population. And people with allergies are not necessarily prone to RA.

> *Because arthritis is an autoimmune condition, it is almost as though arthritics have become allergic to themselves.*

Dear Diary:

Today I ate . . .

Do foods aggravate your arthritis?

Finding the answer isn't very technologically advanced.

The best way to identify potential irritants is to simply keep a food diary and religiously record what you eat and how you feel. Keeping this kind of record is a lot of work. Also, it is difficult to separate foods from other factors that can cause flare ups. Was it the eggplant you ate? Perhaps the yardwork caused this morning's inflammation.

There is no easy answer, but keeping a careful record is the best way to narrow the possibilities.

Eating for Wellness

red meats

fats

salt

caffeine

nightshades

alcohol

junk food

refined flour and rice

all wheat products, from cereal to pasta

additives and preservatives

acidic foods

citrus

pork

smoked or processed meats

dairy products

soda

purines

mixes and prepared foods

canned vegetables

spices

eggs

yeast or fermented foods

Foods Many Arthritis Sufferers Avoid

Recommended Foods for People with Arthritis

vegetables

fruit

fish

fowl

milk

fiber

garlic

water

whole grains

calcium-rich foods

protein, including lean meats

Eating for Wellness

Nightshades are a family of plants which contain solanine, a toxic substance that penetrates the immune barrier and can create painful reactions. Some studies indicate that more than 50 percent of all arthritis patients suffer some toxic effects from nightshades as either the cause of or worsening of their condition.

Solanine-containing Foods Are—

White potatoes   Eggplant   Tomatoes
Red peppers   Tobacco

The most common early symptoms of solanine intolerance are pain and joint stiffness. An elimination diet (systematically eliminating one food at a time, while carefully recording the results in a food diary) may reveal the problem foods. If you eliminate these four foods and tobacco in all forms, your immune system might benefit.

Avoiding these antagonistic foods can be difficult. Some brands of yogurt contain enough potato starch to cause flares. White potato and tomato products are in many packaged foods. Some cheeses contain paprika (derived from peppers). Read the label to know if a food contains one of the culprits. Take your magnifying glass to the grocery store if necessary.

> **Humidity and barometric pressure is usually the culprit in weather-related aggravated arthritis, not the temperature.**

For Crying Out Loud . . .

Caffeine—Caffeine, whether in coffee, tea, soft drinks, chocolate, or medications, whips up your adrenal glands to send forth hormones that make you sensitive to pain.

Nicotine— Smoking nicotine blocks the body's natural pain relievers and stimulates the adrenal glands which makes you more vulnerable to pain. Second-hand smoke may have adverse effects as well.

Climate— An approaching low-pressure system, with a falling barometer, causes an increase in pain and stiffness in some people with arthritis. This has been tested in pressure chambers and found to be true.

Eating for Wellness

Sugar, such as from a soda or candy bar, causes a rise in blood sugar and stimulates the release of insulin. Over time, if you follow a high-sugar meal with a high-sugar snack with another high-sugar meal, your cells become more resistant to the effects of insulin. Its effectiveness decreases, and greater quantities of sugar remain throughout your body, including in the fluid between joints.

The chemical bonding between the sugar in the joints' fluid and the joints' tissues is important to arthritis sufferers. These tissues are joint linings, muscle fibers, tendons, cartilage, and ligaments. This reaction—called glycosylation—goes on continuously and irreversibly in direct proportion to the level of blood sugar. The bonding alters and thus ages the tissues. The more blood sugar, the greater the bonding, the more quickly the joint tissues age.

Turn page for more on sugar. ☞

Sugar, Sugar, Sugar

Some researchers speculate that once this bonding occurs the tissues become more reactive and may bond to other substances circulating in the bloodstream. Other studies indicate that the changes induced by the bonding could cause the immune system to mistake the now-altered tissues—the glycosylated proteins—as foreign and attack them.

Our immune system, though quite impressive, cannot succeed in its ever-vigilant defense of our health unless we keep it in top form. This means not only nourishing it, but protecting it from toxic substances which can include sugar.

Sugar can also reduce the body's ability to convert fats to fatty acids, a necessary job for a healthy immune system. Some studies show as much as a 50-percent reduction in the bacterial-killing power of parts of the immune system in response to a dose of sugar.

Eating for Wellness

Healthy Eating Benefit—

At the very least, by evaluating and improving your eating habits, you may improve your overall health. Not a bad by-product!

———

FYI—

✓   Remember to avoid faddish or extreme diets.

✓   Never stop any medications unless advised by your physician.

✓   Learn all that you can but experiment cautiously.

———

In our modern society, the food industry uses a billion pounds of chemical additives annually. That's 500,000 tons!

Take a half pound of tar and the same quantity of tobacco, and boil them down separately to a thick substance; then simmer them together . . . Apply it to the affected parts.

—Early American "cure" for pain, compiled by Jean Cross

A Real Fish Story . . .

The benefit of fish oils have been a "hot trend" lately. One study reported that it's possible to decrease or stop NSAIDs in patients with rheumatoid arthritis by introducing evening-primrose or fish-oil treatment. They did not suggest the oils replace the drugs, though. This study merely suggested that people tolerate coming off NSAIDs better when they are on long-term fish oil than when they are not. Also, lowering NSAID use would reduce stomach damage.

———

At the University of Washington at Seattle, researchers noted that when they compared hundreds of women with rheumatoid arthritis with those without the disease, there seemed to be a connection between controlling RA and eating baked fish.

Eating for Wellness

Antioxidants

Some scientists speculate that "free radicals" or "oxygen-free radicals," highly unstable chemicals found in the body, play a part in arthritis. These chemicals are believed to develop as a by-product of metabolism—they are the waste products. While most leave the body after the metabolic process is finished, some remain and accumulate. Antioxidants, substances believed to inhibit free-radical reactions, such as betacarotene, vitamin C, vitamin E, and selenium seem to stimulate and strengthen the body's ability to combat disease—arthritis included.

In *How to Beat Arthritis with Immune Power Boosters*, Carlson Wade lists six ways to help keep free radicals under control—

1. Avoid tobacco smoke in all its forms.

2. Keep as far away from air pollution as possible. Take frequent trips to the country or a fresh-air region to cleanse your system.

3. Properly and immediately treat any injury.

4. Say no to anything that is fried, dehydrated, or cured. If you have no alternative, use them at a minimum.

5. Avoid pesticides.

6. Minimize x-rays and ultraviolet radiation.

Free Radicals, and Other Wacky Influences

> *Steam broccoli, spinach, carrots, and cabbage.*

Immune-Boosting Food Strategies

✓ Replace commercial desserts with fresh fruits, especially citrus fruits. Eat sweet potatoes, baked or shredded raw in salads.

✓ Eliminate caffeine-containing beverages.

✓ Enjoy seafood several times a week.

✓ Eat lightly. Steam broccoli, spinach, carrots, and cabbage. Also eat fresh papaya whenever possible.

✓ Sprinkle wheat germ and sunflower seeds on any green salad.

———

GLA (gammalinolenic acid)—

Dr. Lawrence Leventhal in *Annals of Internal Medicine* 1993, reported that GLA reduced the number and severity of tender, swollen joints. The dosage used was very high and it has yet to be approved for treatment of anything. Follow-up trials are being conducted. This might be something to ask your doctor about!

Eating for Wellness

An arthritis sufferer himself, Dr. Collin Dong developed a diet that improved his arthritis. He believes that the average American diet produces nutritional deficiencies. "Just go into food-processing factories, the kitchens of restaurants, hotels, convalescent homes, and sandwich makers and see for yourself how the food is prepared. Chemicals are added to preserve it, color it, and make it taste better. Or go into the slaughterhouses and watch how the meats are prepared and what is done with the leftovers and the various organs. They eventually become luncheon meats, sausages, and the All-American symbol—hot dogs."

Dr. Dong recommends consuming only the basic necessary foods. He doesn't feel the body needs to be overloaded with extras it can't and doesn't need to handle. Here are Dr. Dong's do's and don'ts:

The Arthritic's Cookbook, *by Dr. Collin Dong*

Dr. Dong's Do's

Do eat—

all seafoods

all vegetables including avocados

vegetable oils, particularly safflower and corn

margarine free of milk solids, such as Mazola

egg whites

honey

nuts, sunflower seeds, soybean products

rice of all kinds: brown, white, wild

bread to which nothing in the "don't eat" category
        has been added

tea and coffee

plain soda water

parsley, onion, garlic, bay leaves, salt

any kind of flour

sugar

Eating for Wellness

Don't eat—

meat

dairy products

vinegar or any other acid

chocolate

dry roasted nuts

soft drinks

alcoholic beverages

additives, preservatives, and chemicals, especially

monosodium glutamate (MSG)

Only occasionally eat—

chicken

pasta

Dr. Dong's

Don'ts

But does Dr. Dong's diet work?

Dr. Richard Panush and colleagues at the University of Florida College of Medicine decided to put Dr. Dong's diet to the test. The results do not spell scientific success.

Only two of the 11 patients on the experimental diet greatly improved, but these two, a man and a woman, felt so much better they continued to follow the diet after the experiment was over. Every time they went off it, their arthritis flared. "Without further studies the researchers could not conclude whether the arthritis was modified by the diet or the natural course of the disease."

The man and woman who greatly improved do not care that the results and low success rate do not prove the diet works. They are just glad it works for them.

Eating for Wellness

Diet vs. Nutrition

Do diet and nutrition mean the same thing? The word "nutrition" connotes a more general approach to eating than does the word "diet". Nutrition according to Webster's is "taking in food for living and growing."

It may seem odd in our era of advanced technology, but malnutrition does occur, often because our society eats nutritionally-poor foodstuffs. Advanced nutritional deficiencies can be recognized by the medical profession, but subclinical deficiencies are usually too small to be detected by ordinary means. These are usually multiple in their existence and occur over a period of years bringing on subtle changes in the bones and joints. The result can be degenerative bone and joint disease.

Maintaining a healthy, well-balanced diet is important to everyone, but especially to arthritis patients. You need to take extra care to eat well. The pain from the disease may hinder shopping or cooking. Nausea or other side effects from medicine may kill your appetite. RA patients sometimes have a tendency toward malnutrition. In addition, medications can contribute to malnutrition by depleting your body's vitamins and minerals.

Do diet and nutrition mean the same thing?

Which foods are best with which drugs?

Eat meat, legumes, citrus fruits, dark green leafy vegetables, and whole-grain cereals when taking aspirin and other **NSAIDs**. These foods help reduce stomach irritation and bleeding, and help meet increased nutritional needs for iron, vitamin C, and folic acid.

Avoid alcohol while on **anti-inflammatory drugs**. Alcohol can cause bleeding from the gastrointestinal tract and seems to increase the side effects of anti-inflammatory drugs.

With **corticosteroids**, limit salt and sodium-based seasonings and salty sauces. They can cause water retention and increase the need for calcium, potassium, and certain vitamins. Also avoid foods that taste salty or contain a lot of salt or sodium, including commercial soups, sauces, and even antacids. Softened water can also be a culprit.

Antacids may cause constipation. If constipated, limit antacid use, eat slowly during meals, drink plenty of water, eat prunes, and gradually add fiber to your diet. Also EXERCISE! Taking laxatives can interfere with your body's ability to absorb nutrients. Limit their use. Instead, try the natural methods listed above. Eat a balanced diet.

Eating for Wellness

Hair analysis and nutrition—Hair analysis is not a reliable way to assess nutrition. Dietary history, physical examination, various body measurements, and lab tests are legitimate ways.

———

A balanced diet—A balanced diet can save you money. Money usually spent on tobacco, alcohol, pre-packaged foods, snack foods, junk foods, and red meat can be saved.

———

Sources —

Arthritis Information Magazine, Haymarket Group, Ltd., 45 W. 34th St., New York, NY 10001. (212) 239-0855.

Arthritis Today, Arthritis Foundation, 1330 W. Peachtree St., Atlanta, GA 30309. (800) 933-0032.

"The Prudent Patient," AARP, Fulfillment Section, P.O. Box 2400, Long Beach, CA 90801.

Sears Home Health Care Resource Catalog. (800) 733-7249.

"Laughter—It is infectious and, though intermittent, incurable."

—Ambrose Bierce

References

Arthritis Foundation. *Arthritis in Children.*

Arthritis Foundation. *Arthritis Foundation Aquatic Program.*

Arthritis Foundation. *Arthritis Sourcebook.* Atlanta, GA: Arthritis Foundation. 1996.
Arthritis Today, 9(1-10). 1995.

Arthritis Foundation. (1988). *Guide to Independent Living for People with Arthritis.*
Atlanta, GA: Arthritis Foundation.

Arthritis Foundation. *Health, Life, and Disability Insurance for People with Arthritis.*

Arthritis Foundation. *Living and Loving.*

Arthritis Foundation. *Managing Your Pain.*

Arthritis Foundation. *Travel Tips.*

Arthritis Foundation. *Unproven Remedies.*

Brittan, D. (1996). "A Window on Arthritis." *Technology Review,* 99(7), 12.

Callaghan, J.J. (1996). "A 76-year-old Woman Considering Total Hip Replacement."
JAMA, 276(6), 486.

"Cartilage Care Decreases Risk." *USA Today,* 124(2605), 12. 1995.

Cohen, D. (1995). *Arthritis—Stop Suffering, Start Moving.* New York, NY: Walker and
Co.

Cook, J. (1993). *The Rubicon Dictionary of Positive and Motivational Quotations:
Believed to be the World's Largest Collection of Life-affirming and Inspiring Thoughts and
Sayings.* Newington, CT: Rubicon.

Cough, J. D., Lambert, T., & Miller, D. R. (1996). "The New Thinking on Osteoarthritis."
Patient Care, 30(14), 110.

Delaney, L., Higbee, B., Rao, L., Roth, M., & Yeykal, T. (1993). "Gentle Remedies."
Prevention, 45(7) 6.

Dong, C. H., & Banks, J. (1973). *The Arthritic's Cookbook.* New York, NY: Thomas Y.
Crowell.

Eades, M. D. (1992). *If It Runs in Your Family: Arthritis, Reducing Your Risk.* New York, NY: Bantam Books

Gach, M. R. (1990). *Arthritis Relief at Your Fingertips: The Complete Self-care Guide to Easing Aches and Pains without Drugs.* New York, NY: Reed Warner.

Gadd, I., & Gadd, L. (1985). *Arthritis Alternatives.* New York, NY: Facts on File.

Gleaves, K. (1994). "Get a Grip on Cooking." *Saturday Evening Post, 266*(2), 22.

Gutfeld, G., Sangiorgio, M., & Rao, L. (1993). "Gardening in Full Bloom: Popularity of Activity keeps Growing." *Prevention, 45*(6), 20.

Hawaleshka, D. (1996). "Arthritis Attack: New Research Points to Effective Treatments." *MacLean's, 109*(29), 44.

Henry, S. J. (1996), "Get the Max from your Meds." *Prevention, 48*(9), 72.

Lorig, K., & Fries, J. F. (1995). *The Arthritis Helpbook,* (4th ed.). New York, NY: Addison-Wesley.

Margolis, S., & Flynn, J. A. (1996). *The Johns Hopkins White Papers: Arthritis.* Baltimore, MD: The Johns Hopkins Medical Institutions.

McKenzie, E. C. (1980). *14,000 Quips & Quotes for Writers and Speakers.* Grand Rapids, MI: Baker Book House.

Meyer, M. (1996). "Joint Efforts: You Don't Have to be Sidelined by Osteoarthritis." *Women's Sports & Fitness, 18*(4), 81.

Moyer E. (1993). *Arthritis: Questions You Have—Answers You Need.* Allentown, PA: People's Medical Society.

Morris, David B. (1991). *The Culture of Pain.* University of California Press.

Munson, M. (1994). "Cap Knee Pain." *Prevention, 46*(8), 21.

Munson, M. (1995). "Detective Work Made Easy: How to Finger Trouble with Troubled Hands." *Prevention, 47*(10), 29.

Munson, M. (1995). "New Lean on Life: Postures may Prevent Surgery for Leg Pain." *Prevention, 47*(10), 17.

248

Munson, M. (1995). "Play Away Aches: More Ways to Chase Away Arthritis Pain." *Prevention, 47*(10), 29.

Munson M. (1996). "Tank Heaven: Water Exercise May Unplug Pain." *Prevention, 48*(11), 40.

Park, A. (1996). "Arthritis." *Time, 148*(14), 82.

"Patellar Taping for Relief of Osteoarthritis Pain." *American Family Physician, 50*(3), 676. 1994.

Pisetskey, D. S., & Trien, S. F. (1992). *The Duke University Medical Center Book of Arthritis.* New York, NY: Fawcett Columbine.

Porter, S. F. (1984). *Arthritis Care: A Guide for Patient Education.* Norwalk, CT: Appleton-Centruy-Crofts.

"Prevalence and Impact of Arthritis Among Women—United States," 1989-1991. *MMWR (Morb Mortal Wkly Rep), 44*, 329, 1995.

Ross, P.E. (1993). "Hope for Arthritis Victims." *Forbes, 152*(14), 250.

"Rx for Arthritis Sufferers: Exercise." *Tufts University Diet & Nutrition Letter, 14*(5), 1. 1996.

Sheon, R. P., & Moskowitz, R. W. (1987). *Coping with Arthritis: More Mobility, Less Pain.* New York, NY: McGraw-Hill.

Skerrett, P. J. (1993). "Growing New Cartilage to Fight Arthritis." *Technology Review, 96*(3), 10.

Wade, C. (1989). *How to Beat Arthritis with Immune Power Boosters.* West Nyack, NY: Parker.